KU-611-039

A Guide to Human Helminths

By

ISABEL COOMBS

and

D. W. T. CROMPTON

*W.H.O. Collaborating Centre for Ascariasis,
Department of Zoology,
University of Glasgow, Glasgow G12 8QQ,
Scotland, U.K.*

Taylor and Francis
London • New York • Philadelphia
1991

UK   Taylor & Francis Ltd, 4 John St, London WC1N 2ET

USA   Taylor & Francis Inc., 1900 Frost Rd, Suite 101, Bristol, PA 19007

Copyright © I. Coombs and D. W. T. Crompton, 1991

All rights reserved. No part of this publication may be reproduced, stored in a retrieval system, or transmitted, in any form or by any means, electronic, electrostatic, magnetic tape, mechanical, photocopying, recording or otherwise, without the prior permission of the copyright owner.

British Library Cataloguing in Publication Data

Coombs, Isabel
    Guide to human helminths.
    1. Humans. Parasites
    I. Title   II. Crompton, D. W. T. (David William Thomasson)

    616.96

    ISBN 0-85066-807-7

Library of Congress Cataloging in Publication Data is available.

Cover design by Caroline Archer, cover photograph by Raymond C. Stoddart

Printed in Great Britain by Burgess Science Press, Basingstoke on paper which has a specified pH value on final paper manufacture of not less than 7·5 and is therefore 'acid free'.

Contents

Acknowledgements

We are indebted to the very many scientists whose published work has enabled us to produce this book. Relatively few of them have been cited by name in the text, but this volume would not have appeared without their careful recording of many observations and case histories. Special mention must be made of the inspirational work of Professor P. C. Beaver in the field of human helminthology.

We thank Dr D. I. Gibson, Dr R. A. Bray, Ms E. A. Harris and Mr C. G. Hussey of the Parasitic Worms Section, British Museum (Natural History), for much helpful advice and for access to the B. M.'s Host-Parasite Catalogue. Dr J. Ralph Lichtenfels, Biosystematic Parasitology Laboratory, U.S. Department of Agriculture, Beltsville, Maryland, U.S.A., generously offered much information. Professor S. Pampiglione, Cattedra Di Parassitologia, Universita Degli Studi Di Bologna, Italy, kindly provided much information about human helminth infections in Africa and Europe. Professor D. Bunnag, Faculty of Tropical Medicine, Mahidol University, Bangkok, Thailand, helped us obtain information about trematodes as did Dr E. Pozio, *Trichinella* Reference Centre, Instituto Superiore di Sanita, viale Regina Elena 299, 00161 Roma, Italy, for species of *Trichinella*. Our thanks are also due to Ms M. E. McCulloch and Mr M. L. N. Murthy for their skilful preparation of the typescript. We are most grateful to our publishers for help, support and advice during every stage of the work.

Finally, we invite our readers to send more information, opinions, evidence and suggestions for extending and revising our list of human helminths.

Isabel Coombs and D. W. T. Crompton
Glasgow, October 1990

Introduction

Three hundred and forty two species of helminth, which have been found in association with humans, are listed in this book. 'Helminth' is usually used to describe a worm having an obligatory requirement for a relationship with a living host of a different species. Many of the species of worm listed here undoubtedly deserve the status of parasite; *Ascaris lumbricoides* (p. 153) and *Schistosoma haematobium* (p. 31) are highly prevalent, widely distributed and are recognized in all forms of parasitological literature as parasites of humans. Other species of worm that have occasionally been observed in contact with human tissue may eventually be discarded from this list. For example, a single specimen of *Nybelinia surmenicola* (p. 85) was found attached to a tonsil some hours after the patient had eaten raw squid. A critical discussion of the strength and specificity of different associations between helminths and their hosts has been presented by Prudhoe and Bray (1982).

The theme taken by Norman Stoll for his presidential address to the American Society of Parasitologists, meeting in Boston in December 1946, was to ask and attempt to answer the question 'just how much human helminthiasis is there in the world?' (Stoll, 1947). Estimates of numbers of millions of cases for what Stoll judged to be the common species of helminth parasite of humans are reproduced in Table 1. The values shown in the table have often been derived from data which was not always obtained under ideal conditions. Counting cases relies on appropriate and standardized sampling methods and diagnostic techniques leading to comparable results. Extension of the results from epidemiological surveys to cover an entire country must be based on accurate knowledge of the helminth's distribution in that country. *Ascaris lumbricoides* clearly has an uneven or patchy distribution in many regions (Crompton and Tulley, 1987; Crompton, 1988). Estimates of the numbers of cases of ascariasis in Ghana, for example, would be likely to be misleading if the sampling procedures had been applied only in locations where the prevalence was either high or low (Annan *et al.*, 1986).

Health workers and authorities frequently argue that estimates of numbers of cases for some helminthiases in humans should be regarded as underestimates.

Table 1. Estimates of the numbers of cases (millions) of common human helminthic infections[a]

	Species of helminth	Stoll (1947)	Peters (1978)	Markell and Voge (1981)[c]	Peters and Gilles (1989)
N[b]	Ascaris lumbricoides (p. 153)	644.4	1269	650	1283
N	Dipetalonema perstans (p. 169)	27.0	f	—[d]	65
C	Diphyllobothrium latum (p. 91)	10.4	15		16
N	Dracunculus medinensis (p. 157)	48.3	f	50–80	98
N	Enterobius vermicularis (p. 150)	208.8	353		360
T	Fasciolopsis buski (p. 46)	10.0	g	10	15
N	Filarial worms { Brugia malayi (p. 166) / Wuchereria bancrofti (p. 164)	}189.0	}383	}250[e]	}90
N	Hookworms { Ancylostoma duodenale (p. 133) / Necator americanus (p. 135)	}456.8	}900	}450	}716
N	Loa loa (p. 176)	13.0	f	—	33
N	Mansonella ozzardi (p. 168)	7.0	f	—	15
N	Onchocerca volvulus (p. 168)	19.8	f	20	40
T	Opisthorchis sinensis (= Clonorchis sinensis) (p. 72)	19.0	38	19	28
T	Paragonimus westermani (p. 66)	3.2	g	3.2	5
T	Schistosoma haematobium (p. 31)	39.2	}271	100	78
T	Schistosoma japonicum (p. 32)	46.0		100	69
T	Schistosoma mansoni (p. 33)	29.2		60	57

	Ascaris lumbricoides	Filarial worms	Hookworms	Onchocerca volvulus	Schistosoma spp.	Trichuris trichiura	
	800–1000	250	700–900	30	200	500	Walsh and Warren (1979)
	1000	250	900	30	200	500	Bruer (1982)
	800–1300	90	700–900	20	>200	500	W.H.O. (1986)
	1008 Crompton (1988)	—	—	17.76 WHO (1987a)	—	500–800	Cooper and Bundy (1988)

[b] C, cestode (tapeworm); N, nematode (roundworm); T, trematode (fluke)

[a] In addition, the following estimates of numbers of cases (millions) are also available

		Walsh and Warren (1979)	Bruer (1982)	W.H.O. (1986)	Cooper and Bundy (1988)
N	*Strongyloides stercoralis* (p. 131)	34.9	[h]	35	70
C	*Taeniarhynchus saginatus* (= *Taenia saginata*) (p. 113)	38.9	77	[c]	76
N	*Trichinella spiralis* (p. 117)	27.8	46	—	49
N	*Trichuris trichiura* (p. 119)	355.1	687	350	670
C	*Vampirolepis nana* (= *Hymenolepis nana*) (p. 106)	20.2	39	[c]	29

[c] States that the estimates were supplied by the World Health Organization as of 1975

[d] Cestodiases given as 65 million cases

[e] Assume the estimates for *Loa loa*, *Mansonella ozzardi* and *Onchocerca volvulus* are included in the figure for filarial worms

[f] Other species of filarial nematode (assumed to include these species) are given an estimate of 274 million cases

[g] Other species of trematode (assumed to include these species) are given an estimate of 25 million cases

[h] Other species of non-filarial nematode (assumed to include *Strongyloides stercoralis*) are given an estimate of 85 million cases

Dracunculiasis (48–98 million cases, Table 1) is not a notifiable disease and, since there is no efficacious treatment available, only a small proportion of cases may report to any type of health centre (W.H.O., 1986). Strongyloidiasis (35–56 million cases, Table 1) is not easily diagnosed and autoinfection, causing infections of long duration (Grove, 1986), complicates the estimation of numbers of cases. Nor should it be assumed that a helminthiasis has to be linked to a huge prevalence value and have a worldwide distribution, as is the case for infections described in Table 1, before it has public health significance. Anisakiasis (p. 151), capillariasis (p. 118), angiostrongyliasis (p. 137), fasciolopsiasis (p. 46) and neurocysticercosis (p. 112) are examples of helminthiases having a national or local impact on human health (W.H.O., 1987b).

The entries in this book include species representing the phyla Platyhelminthes (Turbellaria, Digenea, Eucestoda), Nematoda, Nematomorpha and Acanthocephala. The criterion for inclusion in the list is the existence of published evidence describing an actual host-parasite relationship between an individual human being and the worm in question or an association that may point to the existence of such a relationship. The entries encompass worms using humans as definitive and intermediate hosts and cases where the status of the host is uncertain. Associations have not been assigned to such categories as zoonotic, accidental or some other form of infection.

Classification

The helminths considered to infect humans are listed below following a scheme of classification based on the work of Walton and Yokogawa (1972) for the Turbellaria, Yamaguti (1971) for the Digenea, Schmidt (1986) for the Eucestoda, Commonwealth Institute of Helminthology Keys (1974–83) for the Nematoda, Cheng (1973) for the Nematomorpha and Amin (1985) for the Acanthocephala.

PHYLUM PLATYHELMINTHES
CLASS TURBELLARIA

ORDER TRICLADIDA

BIPALIIDAE

Bipalium fuscatum
Bipalium kewense
Bipalium venosum

CLASS TREMATODA (flukes)
SUBCLASS DIGENEA

SCHISTOSOMATIDAE

Schistosoma bovis
Schistosoma haematobium
Schistosoma intercalatum
Schistosoma japonicum
Schistosoma malayensis
Schistosoma mansoni
Schistosoma mattheei
Schistosoma mekongi
Schistosoma rodhaini
Schistosoma spindale
Austrobilharzia terrigalensis
Bilharziella polonica
Gigantobilharzia huttoni
Gigantobilharzia sturniae
Heterobilharzia americana
Orientobilharzia turkestanica
Schistosomatium douthitti
Trichobilharzia brevis
Trichobilharzia ocellata
Trichobilharzia sp. *(T. paoi)*
Trichobilharzia stagnicolae

CLINOSTOMATIDAE

Clinostomum complanatum

CATHYCOTYLIDAE

Prohemistomum vivax

DIPLOSTOMATIDAE

Alaria americana
Alaria marcianae
Diplostomum spathaceum
Fibricola seoulensis

PARAMPHISTOMIDAE

Gastrodiscoides hominis
Watsonius watsoni

FASCIOLIDAE

Fasciola gigantica
Fasciola hepatica
Fasciola indica
Fasciolopsis buski

ECHINOSTOMATIDAE

Echinochasmus japonicus
Echinochasmus jiufoensis
Echinochasmus perfoliatus
Echinoparyphium recurvatum
Echinostoma cinetorchis
Echinostoma echinatum
Echinostoma hortense
Echinostoma ilocanum
Echinostoma macrorchis
Echinostoma malayanum
Echinostoma revolutum
Episthmium caninum
Euparyphium melis
Himasthala muehlensi
Hypoderaeum conoideum

PSILOSTOMIDAE

Psilorchis hominis

LECITHODENDRIIDAE

Phaneropsolus bonnei
Prosthodendrium molenkampi

PLAGIORCHIIDAE

Plagiorchis harinasutai
Plagiorchis javensis
Plagiorchis muris
Plagiorchis philippinensis

CATHAEMASIIDAE

Cathaemasia cabrerai

PHILOPHTHALMIDAE

Philophthalmus lacrymosus
Philophthalmus sp.

DICROCOELIIDAE

Dicrocoelium dendriticum
Dicrocoelium hospes
Eurytrema pancreaticum

PARAGONIMIDAE

Paragonimus africanus
Paragonimus bangkokensis
Paragonimus caliensis
Paragonimus heterotremus
Paragonimus hueit'ungensis
Paragonimus kellicotti
Paragonimus mexicanus
Paragonimus miyazakii
Paragonimus ohirai
Paragonimus philippinensis
Paragonimus pulmonalis
Paragonimus sadoensis
Paragonimus skrjabini
Paragonimus uterobilateralis
Paragonimus westermani
Paragonimus sp.

ACHILLURBAINIIDAE

Achillurbainia nouveli
Achillurbainia recondita
Poikilorchis congolensis

NANOPHYETIDAE

Nanophyetus salmincola salmincola
Nanophyetus salmincola schikhobalowi

OPISTHORCHIDAE

Metorchis albidus
Metorchis conjunctus

Opisthorchis felineus
Opisthorchis guayaquilensis
Opisthorchis noverca
Opisthorchis sinensis
Opisthorchis viverrini
Pseudamphistomum aethiopicum
Pseudamphistomum truncatum

HETEROPHYIDAE

Apophallus donicus

Centrocestus armatus
Centrocestus formosanus

Cryptocotyle lingua

Haplorchis pumilio
Haplorchis taichui
Haplorchis vanissimus
Haplorchis yokogawai

Heterophyes dispar
Heterophyes heterophyes
Heterophyes nocens

Heterophyopsis continua

Metagonimus minutis
Metagonimus yokogawai

Procerovum calderoni
Procerovum varium

Pygidiopsis summa

Stellantchasmus falcatus
Stictodora fuscata

MICROPHALLIDAE

Carneophallus brevicaeca
Microphallus minus

ISOPARORCHIIDAE

Isoparorchis hypselobagri

CLASS CESTOIDEA
SUBCLASS EUCESTODA (strobilate tapeworms)

ORDER TRYPANORHYNCA

TENTACULARIIDAE

Nybelinia surmenicola

ORDER PSEUDOPHYLLIDEA

DIPHYLLOBOTHRIIDAE

Diphyllobothrium cameroni
Diphyllobothrium cordatum
Diphyllobothrium dalliae
Diphyllobothrium dendriticum
Diphyllobothrium elegans
Diphyllobothrium erinaceieuropaei
Diphyllobothrium giljacicum
Diphyllobothrium hians
Diphyllobothrium klebanovskii
Diphyllobothrium lanceolatum
Diphyllobothrium latum
Diphyllobothrium mansoni
Diphyllobothrium mansonoides
Diphyllobothrium minus
Diphyllobothrium nenzi
Diphyllobothrium nihonkaiense

Diphyllobothrium pacificum
Diphyllobothrium scoticum
Diphyllobothrium skrjabini
Diphyllobothrium theileri
Diphyllobothrium tungussicum
Diphyllobothrium ursi
Diphyllobothrium yonagoensis
Diplogonoporus balaenopterae
Diplogonoporus brauni
Diplogonoporus fukuokaensis
Ligula intestinalis
Pyramicocephalus anthocephalus
Schistocephalus solidus

ORDER CYCLOPHYLLIDEA

ANOPLOCEPHALIDAE

Bertiella mucronata
Bertiella studeri
Inermicapsifer madagascariensis
Mathevotaenia symmetrica
Moniezia expansa

DAVAINEIDAE

Raillietina (R.) asiatica
Raillietina (R.) celebensis
Raillietina (R.) madagascariensis

DILEPIDIDAE

Dipylidium caninum

HYMENOLEPIDIDAE

Drepanidotaenia lanceolata
Hymenolepis diminuta
Vampirolepis nana

MESOCESTOIDAE

Mesocestoides lineatus
Mesocestoides variabilis

TAENIIDAE

Echinococcus granulosus
Echinococcus multilocularis
Echinococcus oligarthus
Echinococcus vogeli
Multiceps brauni
Multiceps glomeratus
Multiceps longihamatus
Multiceps multiceps
Multiceps serialis
Taenia crassiceps
Taenia solium
Taenia taeniaeformis
Taeniarhynchus saginatus

PHYLUM NEMATODA (roundworms)

SUPER FAMILY DIOCTOPHYMATOIDEA

DIOCTOPHYMATIDAE

Dioctophyma renale
Eustrongylides sp.

SUPER FAMILY TRICHINELLOIDEA

TRICHINELLIDAE

Trichinella nativa
Trichinella nelsoni
Trichinella spiralis

TRICHURIDAE

Anatrichosoma cutaneum
Aonchotheca philippinensis
Calodium hepaticum
Eucoleus aerophilus
Trichuris suis
Trichuris trichiura
Trichuris vulpis

SUPER FAMILY MERMITHOIDEA

MERMITHIDAE

Agamomermis hominis oris
Agamomermis restiformis
Mermis nigrescens

SUPER FAMILY RHABDITOIDEA

CEPHALOBIDAE

Micronema deletrix
Turbatrix aceti

RHABDITIDAE

Cheilobus quadrilabiatus
Diploscapter coronata
Pelodera strongyloides
Pelodera teres
Rhabditis axei
Rhabditis elongata
Rhabditis inermis
Rhabditis niellyi
Rhabditis pellio
Rhabditis taurica
Rhabditis terricola
Rhabditis sp.

STRONGYLOIDIDAE

Strongyloides canis
Strongyloides cebus
Strongyloides felis
Strongyloides fuelleborni
Strongyloides cf *fuelleborni*
Strongyloides myopotami
Strongyloides papillosus
Strongyloides planiceps
Strongyloides procyonis
Strongyloides ransomi
Strongyloides simiae
Strongyloides stercoralis
Strongyloides westeri

SUPER FAMILY ANCYLOSTOMATOIDEA

ANCYLOSTOMATIDAE

Ancylostoma braziliense
Ancylostoma caninum
Ancylostoma ceylanicum
Ancylostoma duodenale
Ancylostoma japonica
Ancylostoma malayanum
Ancylostoma tubaeforme
Bunostomum phlebotomum
Cyclodontostomum purvisi
Necator americanus
Necator argentinus
Necator suillus
Uncinaria stenocephala

SUPER FAMILY METASTRONGYLOIDEA

ANGIOSTRONGYLIDAE

Parastrongylus cantonensis
Parastrongylus costaricensis
Parastrongylus mackerrasae
Parastrongylus malaysiensis

METASTRONGYLIDAE

Metastrongylus elongatus

SUPER FAMILY STRONGYLOIDEA

CHABERTIIDAE

Oesophagostomum aculeatum
Oesophagostomum apiostomum
Oesophagostomum bifurcum
Oesophagostomum stephanostomum
Ternidens deminutus

SYNGAMIDAE

Mammomonogamus laryngeus
Mammomonogamus nasicola

SUPER FAMILY TRICHOSTRONGYLOIDEA

TRICHOSTRONGYLIDAE

Haemonchus contortus
Marshallagia marshalli
Mecistocirrus digitatus
Nematodirus abnormalis
Ostertagia circumcincta
Ostertagia ostertagi
Trichostrongylus affinus
Trichostrongylus axei
Trichostrongylus brevis
Trichostrongylus calcaratus
Trichostrongylus capricola
Trichostrongylus colubriformis
Trichostrongylus lerouxi
Trichostrongylus orientalis
Trichostrongylus probolurus
Trichostrongylus skrjabini
Trichostrongylus vitrinus

SUPER FAMILY OXYUROIDEA

OXYURIDAE

Enterobius gregorii
Enterobius vermicularis
Syphacia obvelata

SUPER FAMILY ASCARIDOIDEA

ANISAKIDAE

Anisakis simplex
Contracaecum osculatum
Pseudoterranova decipiens

ASCARIDIDAE

Ascaris lumbricoides
Ascaris suum
Baylisascaris procyonis
Lagochilascaris minor

Parascaris equorum
Toxascaris leonina
Toxocara canis
Toxocara cati
Toxocara pteropodis
Toxocara vitulorum

SUPER FAMILY DRACUNCULOIDEA

DRACUNCULIDAE

Dracunculus medinensis

PHILOMETRIDAE

Philometra sp.

SUPER FAMILY GNATHOSTOMATOIDEA

GNATHOSTOMATIDAE

Gnathostoma doloresi
Gnathostoma hispidum
Gnathostoma spinigerum

SUPER FAMILY PHYSALOPTEROIDEA

PHYSALOPTERIDAE

Physaloptera caucasica
Physaloptera transfuga

SUPER FAMILY RICTULARIOIDEA

RICTULARIIDAE

Rictularia sp.

SUPER FAMILY THELAZIOIDEA

THELAZIIDAE

Thelazia californiensis
Thelazia callipaeda

SUPER FAMILY SPIRUROIDEA

GONGYLONEMATIDAE

Gongylonema pulchrum

SPIROCERCIDAE

Spirocerca lupi

SUPER FAMILY ACUARIOIDEA

ACUARIIDAE

Cheilospirura sp.

SUPER FAMILY FILARIOIDEA

ONCHOCERCIDAE

Wuchereria bancrofti
Wuchereria lewisi
Brugia beaveri
Brugia guyanensis
Brugia malayi
Brugia pahangi
Brugia timori
Onchocerca volvulus
Mansonella (Mansonella) ozzardi
Mansonella (Esslingeria) perstans
Mansonella semiclarum
Mansonella (Esslingeria) streptocerca
Dipetalonema arbuta
Dipetalonema sprenti
Microfilaria bolivarensis
Microfilaria (Mansonella) rodhaini
Meningonema peruzzii
Setaria equina
Dirofilaria (D.) immitis
Dirofilaria (Nochtiella) repens
Dirofilaria spectans
Dirofilaria (Nochtiella) striata
Dirofilaria (Nochtiella) tenuis
Dirofilaria (Nochtiella) ursi
Loa loa

PHYLUM NEMATOMORPHA (horsehair worms)

GORDIIDAE

Gordius aquaticus
Gordius chilensis
Gordius gesneri
Gordius inesae
Gordius ogatai
Gordius perronciti
Gordius reddyi
Gordius robustus
Gordius setiger
Gordius skorikowi

CHORDODIDAE

Chordodes capensis
Neochordodes colombianus
Parachordodes alpestris
Parachordodes pustulosus
Parachordodes raphaelis
Parachordodes tolosanus
Parachordodes violaceus
Parachordodes wolterstorffii
Paragordius areolatus
Paragordius cinctus
Paragordius esavianus
Paragordius tricuspidatus
Paragordius varius
Pseudogordius tanganyikae

PHYLUM ACANTHOCEPHALA (thorny-headed worms)
CLASS ARCHIACANTHOCEPHALA

MONILIFORMIDAE

Moniliformis moniliformis

OLIGACANTHORHYNCHIDAE

Macracanthorhynchus hirudinaceus
Macracanthorhynchus ingens

CLASS PALAEACANTHOCEPHALA

ECHINORHYNCHIDAE

Acanthocephalus rauschi
Pseudoacanthocephalus bufonis

POLYMORPHIDAE

Bolbosoma sp.
Corynosoma strumosum

List of
Human Helminths

The entries in this list are presented, whenever the information permits, in a standard format which requires some explanation and interpretation. The information for *Taeniarhynchus saginatus* (p. 113), which is reproduced below, provides an example of a typical entry.

Taeniarhynchus saginatus[1] (Goeze, 1782) Weinland, 1858

S: *Taenia saginata*

DH: MAN[2]

IH: Many species of herbivorous mammal including domesticated cattle and *Rangifer rangifer* (reindeer)

GD: Worldwide where humans and cattle are associated

---

[1] Scientific name for the species. The validity of the name is based on consultation of a considerable volume of systematic and taxonomic literature together with advice from colleagues at the British Museum (Natural History). A full appraisal of synonyms and priorities is beyond the scope of this book; the scientific names given here have been chosen for convenience and with a view to improving communication. There are still cases where much work will need to be done before the taxonomy and nomenclature of a helminth's genus and species will achieve a satisfactory and agreed position. The case of the confusion around the name of the genus *Dipetalonema* provides an example of the problems awaiting solution (Muller, 1987).

[2] MAN (in capital letters) is used to indicate that the host status (**DH, H, IH,** or **PH** – for definitions see below) has been established or can be assumed. Man (in lower case letters) is used either when the host status is unresolved or when the helminth in question does not appear to attain sexual maturity.

LM: Adult worm located in small intestine, occasionally other sites; cysticerci, identified as *T. saginatus*, have been found in human tissue

ND: Taeniasis due to *Taenia saginata*

TM: Ingestion of cysticercus in raw or undercooked beef

Pawlowski, Z. S. and Schultz, M. G., 1972, Taeniasis and cysticercosis (*Taenia saginata*).
Advances in Parasitology, **10**, 269–343.[3]

Abbreviations for entries

DH, definitive host(s). A definitive host is defined as a species of host in which
the helminth species is known or is assumed to attain sexual maturity.

H, host. In some cases, for example the life histories of species of Nematomorpha discussed by Cappucci (1976), the usual concepts of definitive
and intermediate host do not apply and it seems more appropriate to
refer to the host.

IH, intermediate host(s), sometimes subdivided into first (**IH1**) and second
(**IH2**) intermediate hosts. An intermediate host is defined as a species of
host in which the helminth species is known or is assumed to develop,
but in which sexual maturity is not attained.

PH, paratenic host(s). A paratenic host is defined as a species of host which
ensures or enhances the transmission of the helminth species to the
definitive host, but is not necessary for the development or sexual
maturation of the helminth species.

GD, geographical distribution. The names for continents and countries,
based on the tables published by the Centers for Disease Control,
Atlanta, Georgia, U.S.A. (1985), have been used to point readers to the
geographical distribution of the helminths (Table 2). The term "worldwide", sometimes used in conjunction with a climatic term, indicates
that a helminth species is widely distributed either in human or in non-
human hosts. The distribution of helminths that are considered to be
restricted to a region, for example *Parastrongylus costaricensis* (p. 138) is
shown as follows "The Americas (Costa Rica, Nicaragua, Panama,
Peru)".

---

[3] A reference chosen to offer a general introduction to the human host-helminth relationship in
question. In cases where the presence of the helminth in humans appears to be rare, the reference
usually includes a convincing description of a case history.

Table 2. The continental regions and countries of the world (based on information given CDC, 1985)

AFRICA

Algeria	Ghana	Reunion (France)
Angola	Guinea	Rwanda
Benin	Guinea-Bissau	Saint Helena (U.K.)
Botswana	Ivory Coast	Sao Tome and Princi
Burkina Faso	Kenya	Senegal
Burundi	Lesotho	Seychelles
Cameroon	Liberia	Sierra Leone
Canary Islands (Spain)	Libyan Arab Jamahiriya	Somalia
Cape Verde	Madagascar	South Africa
Central African Republic	Madeira (Portugal)	Sudan
Chad	Malawi	Swaziland
Comoros	Mali	Tanzania, United
Congo	Mauritania	Republic of
Djibouti	Mauritius	Togo
Egypt	Morocco	Tunisia
Equatorial Guinea	Mozambique	Uganda
Ethiopia	Namibia	Zaire
Gabon	Niger	Zambia
Gambia	Nigeria	Zimbabwe

THE AMERICAS

Argentina	Ecuador	Nicaragua
Belize	El Salvador	Panama
Bermuda (U.K.)	Falkland Islands (U.K.)	Paraguay
Bolivia	French Guiana	Peru
Brazil	Greenland (Denmark)	St Pierre and
Canada	Guatemala	Miquelon (France)
Chile	Guyana	Surinam
Colombia	Honduras	United States of Amer
Costa Rica	Mexico	Uruguay
Cuba		Venezuela

ASIA

Afghanistan	Korea, Democratic	Philippines
Bahrain	People's Republic of	Qatar
Bangladesh	(North)	Ryukyu Islands (Japar
Bhutan	Korea, Republic of (South)	Saudi Arabia
Brunei Darussalam	Kuwait	Singapore
China	Laos People's Democratic	Sri Lanka
Cyprus	Republic	Syrian Arab Republic
Hong Kong (U.K.)	Lebanon	Taiwan
India	Macao (Portugal)	Thailand
Indonesia	Malaysia	Turkey
Iran, Islamic Republic of	Maldives	United Arab Emirates
Iraq	Mongolia	Viet Nam
Israel	Myanmar [= Burma]	Yemen
Japan	Nepal	Yemen, Democra
Jordan	Oman	
Kampuchea	Pakistan	

Table 2 (*contd*)

THE CARIBBEAN

Bahamas
Cayman Islands (U.K.)
Greater Antilles:
  Dominican Republic,
  Haiti, Jamaica,
  Puerto Rico (U.S.)
Lesser Antilles:
  Netherlands Antilles:
    Aruba, Bonaire,
    Curacao
  Trinidad and Tobago

Leeward Islands:
  Anguilla (U.K.),
  Antigua and Barbuda,
  Guadeloupe (France),
  Montserrat (U.K.),
  Saint Christopher
    (St Kitts)
  and Nevis (U.K.),
  Saint Martin (Fr. & Neth.)
  Virgin Islands, British
  Virgin Islands (U.S.)

Windward Islands:
  Barbados, Dominica,
  Grenada, Martinique
    (France),
  Saint Lucia,
  Saint Vincent and
  the Grenadines

EUROPE

Albania
Andorra
Austria
Azores (Portugal)
Belgium
Bulgaria
Czechoslovakia
Denmark
Faroe Islands (Denmark)
Finland
France
Germany
Gibraltar (U.K.)

Greece
Hungary
Iceland
Ireland
Italy
Liechtenstein
Luxembourg
Malta
Monaco
Netherlands
Norway
Poland
Portugal

Romania
San Marino
Spain
Sweden
Switzerland
Union of Soviet
  Socialist Republics
United Kingdom (with
  Channel Islands and
  Isle of Man)
Yugoslavia

OCEANIA

Australia
Christmas Island
  (Australia)
Fiji
French Polynesia (Tahiti)
Guam (U.S.)
Kiribati
Nauru

New Caledonia (France)
New Zealand
Niue (New Zealand)
Northern Mariana Islands
Pacific Islands, Trust
  Territory of the USA
Papua New Guinea
Pitcairn (U.K.)

Samoa
Samoa, American (U.S.)
Solomon Islands
Tonga
Tuvalu
Vanuatu
Wake Island (U.S.)

LM, location(s) of the helminth species in the human host. Usually in cases where the occurrence of a helminth species in association with a human host appears to be rare, a quotation is given from a primary source in the published literature.

ND, name of the disease recommended by CIOMS/WHO (1987). The names of helminths in the CIOMS/WHO list do not always correspond with our choice of valid scientific names.

S,   synonym or name judged to be in common usage.

TM,   mode(s), actual or assumed, of transmission to the human host.

The entries in this book include technical terms which describe developmental or life history stages of the species of helminth concerned. We have set out below definitions of these terms as we have used them for the taxonomic groups mentioned in the classification given on page 5. Further discussion of these terms and many examples of their use are given by Schmidt and Roberts (1981).

Cercaria

A cercaria is an aquatic, free-living, dispersive stage in the life history of a trematode belonging to the subclass Digenea. Cercariae, which are short-lived and do not feed, represent the end-product of asexual reproduction in the molluscan host and in most species they give rise to metacercariae. Cercariae of some species of the super family Strigeoidea develop into mesocercariae while those of the super family Schistosomatoidea develop to the adult fluke after invasion of the definitive host without transformation to mesocercarial or metacercarial stages.

Coenurus

A coenurus is a bladder stage of a larval cestode of certain species of the order Cyclophyllidea. Multiple protoscolices bud off from the inner germinal layer of the bladder and these are infective when swallowed by susceptible definitive hosts.

Cystacanth

A cystacanth, which is readily recognized by its inverted, hook-bearing proboscis or attachment organ, is the stage formed on the completion of the development of an acanthocephalan worm in the body cavity of its arthropod intermediate host. When intermediate hosts harbouring cystacanths are swallowed by susceptible definitive and paratenic hosts, sexually mature adults develop in the small intestines of definitive hosts and juvenile forms are subsequently found encapsulated in the viscera of paratenic hosts.

Cysticercoid

A cysticercoid is the solid stage formed in the body cavity when the development of species of cestode belonging to the order Cyclophyllidea is completed in an invertebrate intermediate host. A cysticercoid contains an invaginated scolex or attachment organ which usually bears suckers and hooks. Ingestion of cysticercoids by a susceptible definitive host leads to the establishment of an infection of sexually mature tapeworms in the alimentary tract.

Cysticercus

A cysticercus is the bladder stage formed in the body cavity or organs when the development of species of cestode belonging to the order Cyclophyllidea is completed in a vertebrate intermediate host. A cysticercus contains an invaginated and introverted scolex or attachment organ which usually bears hooks and suckers. Ingestion of cysticerci by susceptible definitive hosts leads to the establishment of sexually mature tapeworms in the alimentary tract.

Hydatid cyst

A *unilocular* hydatid cyst is the site of asexual reproduction in the cyclophyllidean cestode *Echinococcus granulosus* (p. 108). Cysts are found in and between the internal organs of mammalian intermediate hosts including humans. Each cyst develops from the larva (oncosphere) contained within an egg and, as the cyst grows, millions of protoscolices (stages infective to susceptible definitive hosts) are produced by budding from the tissues lining the inside of the cyst wall. The development pattern of *Echinococcus multilocularis* (p. 108) is similar except that the hydatid cyst is described as *multilocular* because it exhibits extensive endogenous budding. Ingestion of protoscolices by a susceptible definitive host leads to the establishment of sexually mature tapeworms in the small intestine.

Mesocercaria

A mesocercaria is a morphologically distinct, prolonged intermediate stage in the development of a cercaria to a metacercaria during the life history of a number of species of trematode belonging to the digenean family Diplostomatidae. Mesocercariae become established when cercariae invade susceptible intermediate hosts; they subsequently give rise to metacercariae as the life histories of their species progress.

Metacercaria

A metacercaria is the encysted stage in the life history of a trematode belonging to the subclass Digenea. Metacercariae are usually formed directly from cercariae and are located on or in the appropriate second intermediate host. Exceptions occur in the life histories of species of Fasciolidae and Paramphistomatidae in which the metacercariae are found encysted on vegetation. Typically, ingestion of metacercariae by a susceptible definitive host leads to the establishment of an infection of sexually mature flukes.

Microfilaria

A microfilaria is the minute (approx. 250 μm long), first-stage larva or juvenile in the life history of a species of nematode of the order Filarioidea. Microfilariae are detected in the body fluids and tissues of definitive hosts after release from their parent female worms. A sheathed microfilaria is encased in the thin egg shell which has become stretched and elongated. An unsheathed microfilaria is naked having escaped from the egg shell. Microfilariae function as dispersive stages and are responsible for the infection of the intermediate host.

Plerocercoid

A plerocercoid is the stage between a procercoid and an adult in the life history of a species of cestode belonging to the order Pseudophyllidea. Plerocercoids, which are usually found in the body cavities and tissues of second intermediate hosts, give rise to sexually mature tapeworms in the alimentary tract after ingestion by a susceptible definitive host. A plerocercoid possesses an attachment organ or scolex and many of the features of an adult tapeworm, but functional genitalia are absent and segmentation is usually lacking or poorly developed.

Procercoid

A procercoid is the stage formed on completion of the development of a pseudophyllidean cestode in its first intermediate host. Ingestion of procercoids by susceptible second intermediate hosts gives rise to plerocercoids.

Sparganum

A sparganum is the name usually reserved for the plerocercoid stage of species of pseudophyllidean cestode of the genus *Spirometra*.

Information about concepts such as prevalence, intensity and other ecological and epidemiological terms of relevance to helminthology is to be found in a report prepared by a working party of the American Society of Parasitologists (Margolis *et al.*, 1982).

REFERENCES

Amin, O. M., 1985, Classification. In Crompton, D. W. T. and Nickol, B. B. (Eds), *Biology of the Acanthocephala*, pp. 27–72, Cambridge University Press.

Annan, A., Crompton, D. W. T., Walters, D. E. and Arnold, S., 1986, An investigation of the prevalence of intestinal parasites in preschool children in Ghana, *Parasitology*, **92**, 209–217.

Bruer, J., 1982, The great neglected diseases. *R.F. Illustrated.* The Rockefeller Foundation, June 1982.

Cappucci, D. T., 1976, *The Biology of* Gordius robustus *Leidy with a Host List and Summary of the Public Health Importance of the Gordioidea.* PhD Dissertation: University of California, San Francisco. (University Microfilms International, Ann Arbor, Michigan).

C.D.C., 1985, *Health Information for International Travel*, Atlanta, Georgia: U.S. Department of Health and Human Services, Centers for Disease Control.

Cheng, T. C., 1973, *General Parasitology*, New York and London: Academic Press.

C.I.H. Keys, 1974–83, *Commonwealth Institute of Helminthology Keys to the Nematode*

Parasites of Vertebrates edited by R. C. Anderson, A. G. Chabaud and S. M. Willmott, Tarnham Royal, Bucks, U.K.: Commonwealth Agricultural Bureaux, in 10 parts.

C.I.O.M.S./W.H.O., 1987, *International Nomenclature of Diseases. II. Infectious Diseases. Part 4: Parasitic Diseases*. Geneva, Switzerland: World Health Organization.

Cooper, E. S. and Bundy, D. A. P., 1988, *Trichuris* is not trivial, *Parasitology Today*, **4**, 301–306.

Crompton, D. W. T., 1988, The prevalence of ascariasis, *Parasitology Today*, **4**, 162–169.

Crompton, D. W. T. and Tulley, J. J., 1987, How much ascariasis is there in Africa? *Parasitology Today*, **3**, 123–127.

Grove, D. I., 1986, Replicating helminth parasites of man, *Parasitology Today*, **2**, 107–111.

Margolis, L., Esch, G. W., Holmes, J. C., Kuris, A. M. and Schad, G. A., 1982, The use of ecological terms in parasitology. (Report of an *ad hoc* committee of the American Society of Parasitologists), *Journal of Parasitology*, **68**, 131–133.

Markell, E. K. and Voge, M., 1981, *Medical Parasitology*, 5th edition, London and Philadelphia: W. B. Saunders Company.

Muller, R., 1987, A *Dipetalonema* by any other name, *Parasitology Today*, **3**, 358–359.

Peters, W., 1978, Medical aspects – comments and discussion II. In: *The Relevance of Parasitology to Human Welfare* edited by A. E. R. Taylor and R. Muller, Oxford: Blackwell Scientific Publications.

Peters, W. and Gilles, H. M., 1989, *A Colour Atlas of Tropical Medicine and Parasitology*, 3rd edition, London: Wolfe Medical Publications Ltd.

Prudhoe, S. and Bray, R. A., 1982, *Platyhelminth Parasites of the Amphibia*. British Museum (Natural History), Oxford University Press.

Schmidt, G. D., 1986, *Handbook of Tapeworm Identification*, Boca Raton, Florida: CRC Press Inc.

Schmidt, G. D. and Roberts, L. S., 1981, *Foundations of Parasitology*, 2nd edition, St Louis, Toronto, London: The C. V. Mosby Company.

Stoll, N. R., 1947, This wormy world, *Journal of Parasitology*, **33**, 1–18.

Walsh, J. A. and Warren, K. S., 1979, Selective primary health care, *New England Journal of Medicine*, **301**, 967–974.

Walton, B. C. and Yokogawa, M., 1972, Terrestrial turbellarians (Tricladida: Bipaliidae) as pseudoparasites of man, *Journal of Parasitology*, **58**, 444–446.

W.H.O., 1986, Major parasitic infections: a global review, *World Health Statistics Quarterly*, **39**, 145–160.

W.H.O., 1987*a*, Onchocerciasis, *Technical Report Series 752*, Geneva: World Health Organization.

W.H.O., 1987*b*, Prevention and control of intestinal parasitic infections. *Technical Report Series 749*, Geneva: World Health Organization.

Yamaguti, S., 1971, *Synopsis of Digenetic Trematodes of Vertebrates*, Tokyo, Japan: Keigaku Publishing Co.

In addition to the references cited above and those given with the entries for individual species of helminth, much valuable information about human helminths and their investigation has been drawn from the records maintained by the staff of the Parasitic Worms Section, BM(NH), the Index-Catalogue of Medical and Veterinary Zoology, U.S. Department of Agriculture and from the following sources:

Ash, L. R. and Orihel, T. C., 1989, *Atlas of Human Parasitology*, 3rd edition, Chicago: American Society of Clinical Parasitologists.

Beaver, P. C., 1969, The nature of visceral larva migrans, *Journal of Parasitology*, **55**, 3–12.

Beaver, P. C. and Jung, R. C. (eds), 1985, *Animal Agents and Vectors of Human Disease*, 5th edition, Philadelphia: Lea and Febiger.

Beaver, P. C., Jung, R. C. and Cupp, E. W., 1984, *Clinical Parasitology*, 9th edition, Philadelphia: Lea and Febiger.

Bell, J. C., Palmer, S. R. and Payne, J. M., 1988, *The Zoonoses*, London, Baltimore, Melbourne, Auckland: Edward Arnold.

Geerts, S., Kumar, V. and Brandt, T. (eds), 1987, *Helminth Zoonoses*, Dordrecht, Boston, Lancaster: Martinus Nijhoff Publishers.

Hillyer, G. V. and Hopla, C. E., 1982, *CRC Handbook Series in Zoonoses. Section C, Parasitic Zoonoses, III*, Boca Raton, Florida: CRC Press Inc.

Hubbert, W. T., McCulloch, D. V. M. and Schnurrenberger, P. R. (eds), 1975, *Diseases Transmitted from Animals to Man*, 6th edition, Springfield, Illinois, U.S.A.: Charles C. Thomas.

Jacobs, L. and Arambulo, P. (eds), 1982, *CRC Handbook Series in Zoonoses. Section C, Parasitic Zoonoses, I*, Boca Raton, Florida: CRC Press Inc.

Rollinson, D. and Simpson, A. J. G. (eds), 1987, *The Biology of Schistosomes*, New York and London: Academic Press.

Schultz, M. G. (ed.), 1982, *CRC Handbook Series in Zoonoses. Section C, Parasitic Zoonoses, II*, Boca Raton, Florida: CRC Press Inc.

Soulsby, E. J. L., 1982, *Helminths, Arthropods and Protozoa of Domesticated Animals*, 7th edition, London: Bailliere Tindall.

W.H.O., 1980, *Manual of Basic Techniques for a Health Laboratory*, Geneva, Switzerland: World Health Organization.

PLATYHELMINTHES

TURBELLARIA

  TRICLADIDA

  BIPALIIDAE

Bipalium fuscatum Stimpson, 1857

H: Man; adult worms are terrestrial, free-living animals

GD: Asia (Japan); worm widely distributed in humid tropical regions

LM: "... coughed up a 10 cm-long flatworm ... presumed ... present in the respiratory tract, probably in the nasopharynx ..."

TM: Unresolved

Walton, B. C. and Yokogawa, M., 1972, Terrestrial turbellarians (Tricladida: Bipaliidae) as pseudoparasites of man. *Journal of Parasitology*, **58**, 444–446.

Bipalium kewense Mosely, 1878

H: Man; adult worms are terrestrial, free-living animals

GD: Asia (Japan); worm widely distributed in humid tropical regions

LM: "... a diaper with a fresh stool containing an active flatworm ... the mother who said it passed with the stool."

TM: Unresolved

Walton, B. C. and Yokogawa, M., 1972, Terrestrial turbellarians (Tricladida: Bipaliidae) as pseudoparasites of man. *Journal of Parasitology*, **58**, 444–446.

Bipalium venosum Kaburaki, 1922

H: Man; adult worms are terrestrial, free-living animals

GD: Asia (Japan); worm widely distributed in humid tropical regions

LM: "... a very active blood-covered flatworm, approximately 6 cm in length, was passed during defecation."

TM: Unresolved

Walton, B. C. and Yokogawa, M., 1972, Terrestrial turbellarians (Tricladida: Bipaliidae) as pseudoparasites of man. *Journal of Parasitology*, **58**, 444–446.

TREMATODA

DIGENEA

SCHISTOSOMATIDAE

Schistosoma bovis (Sonsino, 1876) Blanchard, 1895

DH: MAN; domesticated and wild species of ruminant and herbivorous mammal

IH: Species of *Bulinus* including *B. africanus* and *B. truncatus*, also *Planorbarius metidjensis* (snails)

GD: Africa (Kenya, Niger, Senegal, South Africa, Uganda, Zaire, Zimbabwe); Europe (Italy); widespread in domesticated ruminants in tropics

LM: Eggs identified in stools implying presence of adults in mesenteric blood vessels following cercarial migration

ND: Schistosomiasis due to *Schistosoma bovis*
          Cercarial dermatitis due to *Schistosoma bovis*

TM: Skin penetration by cercaria in contaminated fresh water

Chunge, R., Katsivo, M., Kok, P., Wamivea, M. and Kinoti, S., 1986, *Schistosoma bovis* in human stools in Kenya. *Transactions of the Royal Society of Tropical Medicine and Hygiene*, **80**, 849.

Schistosoma haematobium (Bilharz, 1852) Weinland, 1858

DH: MAN; species of non-human primate including *Cercopithecus pygerethrus* (vervet monkey), domesticated sheep and *Arvicanthus niloticus* (nile rat)

IH: Species of *Bulinus* including *B. africanus*, *B. truncatus* and *B. senegalensis* (snails)

GD: Africa (34 countries); Asia (Iran, Iraq, Jordan, Syrian Arab Republic)

LM: Adults usually in veins of urinary bladder following cercarial migration

ND: Schistosomiasis due to *Schistosoma haematobium*

TM: Skin penetration by cercaria in contaminated fresh water

Rollinson, D. and Southgate, V. R., 1987, The genus *Schistosoma*: a taxonomic appraisal. In *The Biology of Schistosomes*, edited by D. Rollinson and A. J. G. Simpson (London and New York: Academic Press) pp. 1–49.

Schistosoma intercalatum Fisher, 1934

DH: MAN; experimentally in non-human primates, sheep, goats, cattle, gerbils and hamsters

IH: Species of *Bulinus* including *B. forskalii* and *B. globosus* (snails)

GD: Africa (Cameroon, Central African Republic, Equatorial Guinea, Gabon, Zaire)

LM: Adults in mesenteric blood vessels following cercarial migration

ND: Schistosomiasis due to *Schistosoma intercalatum*

TM: Skin penetration by cercaria in contaminated fresh water

Corachan, M., Mas, R., Palacin, A., Romero, R., Mondelo, F. and Pujol, M., 1987, Autochthonous case of *Schistosoma intercalatum* from Equatorial Guinea. *American Journal of Tropical Medicine and Hygiene*, **36**, 343–344.

Schistosoma japonicum Katsurada, 1904

DH: MAN; many species of domesticated and wild mammal

IH: Species of *Oncomelania* including *O. formosana*, *O. hupensis*, *O. noso-phora* and *O. quadrasi* (snails)

GD: Asia (China, Indonesia, Japan, Malaysia, Philippines, Thailand)

LM: Adults in mesenteric blood vessels following cercarial migration

ND: Schistosomiasis due to *Schistosoma japonicum*

TM: Skin penetration by cercaria in contaminated fresh water

Olveda, R. M. and Domingo, E. O., 1987, Schistosomiasis japonica. In *Clinical Tropical Medicine and Communicable Diseases* edited by A. A. F. Mahmoud (London and Philadelphia: Bailliere Tindall) pp. 397–417.

Schistosoma malayensis Greer, Ow-Yang and Yong, 1988

DH: MAN; *Rattus muelleri* and *R. tiomanicus* (rats), mouse (experimental)

IH: Species of *Robertsiella* including *R. gismanni* and *R. kaporensis* (snails)

GD: Asia (Malaysia)

LM: Ten cases diagnosed as schistosomiasis have been reported on the basis of eggs found in tissues including the liver

ND: Schistosomiasis due to *Schistosoma malayensis*

TM: Skin penetration by cercaria in contaminated fresh water

Greer, G. J., Ow-Yang, C. K. and Hoi-Senh Yong, 1988, *Schistosoma malayensis* n.sp.: A *Schistosoma japonicum*—complex schistosoma from peninsular Malaysia. *Journal of Parasitology*, **74**, 471–480.

Schistosoma mansoni Sambon, 1907

DH: MAN; many domesticated and wild species of mammal

IH: Species of *Biomphalaria* including *B. alexandrina, B. glabrata* and *B. pfeifferi* (snails)

GD: Africa (39 countries); The Americas (Brazil, Surinam, Venezuela); Asia (Oman, Saudi Arabia, Yemen); The Caribbean (Antigua, Dominican Republic, Guadeloupe, Martinique, Montserrat, Puerto Rico, Saint Lucia)

LM: Adults in mesenteric blood vessels following cercarial migration

ND: Schistosomiasis due to *Schistosoma mansoni*

TM: Skin penetration by cercaria in contaminated fresh water

Doumenge, J. P., Mott, K. E., Cheung, C., Villenave, D., Chapuis, O., Perrin, M. F. and Reauo-Thomas, G., 1987, *Atlas of the Global Distribution of Schistosomiasis* (Geneva: World Health Organization and University of Bordeaux Press).

Schistosoma mattheei Veglia and Le Roux, 1929

DH: MAN; domesticated and wild species of ruminant mammal

IH: Species of *Bulinus* including *B. africanus* and *B. globosus* (snails)

GD: Africa (South Africa, Zambia, Zimbabwe)

LM: Adults assumed to be in mesenteric blood vessels following cercarial migration; "Rectal snips and biopsy showed that many ova penetrated the tissues".

ND: Schistosomiasis due to *Schistosoma mattheei*
Cercarial dermatitis due to *Schistosoma mattheei*

TM: Skin penetration by cercaria in contaminated fresh water

Hira, P. R., 1975, Observations on *Schistosoma mattheei* Veglia and Le Roux, 1929 infections in man in Zambia. *Annales de la Societe Belge de Medicine Tropicale*, **55**, 633–642.

Schistosoma mekongi Voge, Bruckner and Bruce, 1978

DH: MAN; domesticated dog

IH: *Tricula aperta* (snail)

GD: Asia (Cambodia, Laos, Thailand)

LM: Presumably adults in mesenteric blood vessels following cercarial migration

ND: Schistosomiasis due to *Schistosoma mekongi*

TM: Skin penetration by cercaria in contaminated fresh water

Duong, T. H., Arbeille, B., Karagirwa, A., Lorette, G. and Combescot, Ch., 1986, Schistosomiasis mekongi along the Mekong and its affluents Mun and Tonle Sap. Report of two cases observed in Tours. *Bulletin Societe Pathologie Exotique*, **79**, 222–228.

Schistosoma rodhaini Brumpt, 1931

DH: MAN; domesticated dog, species of rodent

IH: Species of *Biomphalaria* including *B. pfeifferi* and *B. sudanica* (snails)

GD: Africa (Zaire)

LM: Presumably venous blood vessels

ND: Schistosomiasis due to *Schistosoma rodhaini*

TM: Skin penetration by cercaria in contaminated fresh water

D'Haenens, G. and Santele, A., 1955, Sur un cas humain de *Schistosoma rodhaini* trouve aux environs d'Elisabethville. *Annales de la Societe Belge de Medicine Tropicale*, **35**, 497–498.

Schistosoma spindale Montgomery, 1906

DH: Man; many species of domesticated and wild mammal

IH: *Indoplanorbis exustus* (snail)

GD: Asia (India, Indonesia, Malaysia, Sri Lanka, Thailand, Vietnam)

LM: Cercaria in skin

ND: Cercarial dermatitis due to *Schistosoma spindale*

TM: Skin penetration by cercaria in contaminated fresh water

Harinasuta, C., 1971, Human and non-human schistosomiasis in Thailand. *The Proceedings of the 12th Pacific Science Congress*, Canberra, Australia. 1, Section A. Symposium A9 p. 202. Abstract.

Austrobilharzia terrigalensis Johnston, 1917

DH: Man; many species of wading bird, sea bird and waterfowl

IH: Species of *Littorina* including *L. pintado* and *L. planaxis* (snails)

GD: Oceania (Australia); helminth widely distributed in species of aquatic bird

LM: Cercaria in skin

ND: Cercarial dermatitis due to *Austrobilharzia terrigalensis*

TM: Skin penetration by cercaria in contaminated brackish or sea water

Rhode, K., 1977, The bird schistosome *Austrobilharzia terrigalensis* from the Great Barrier Reef, Australia. *Zeitschrift fur Parasitenkunde*, **52**, 39.

Bilharziella polonica (Kowalewski, 1895) Looss, 1899

DH: Man; many species of wading bird, sea bird and waterfowl

IH: Species of *Coretus, Planorbis, Physopsis* and *Spirolina* (snails)

GD: Europe (Finland; USSR, Siberia, Turkestan, Urals); helminth widely distributed in species of aquatic bird

LM: Cercaria in skin

ND: Cercarial dermatitis due to *Bilharziella polonica*

TM: Skin penetration by cercaria in contaminated water

Pirila, V. and Wikgren, B. J., 1957, Cases of swimmers' itch in Finland. *Acta Dermato-Venereologica*, **37**, 140–148.

Gigantobilharzia huttoni (Leigh, 1953) Leigh, 1955

DH: Man; *Pelecanus occidentalis* (brown pelican) and *P. erythrorhynchos* (white pelican)

IH: *Haminoea antillarum guadalupensis* (marine snail)

GD: The Americas (USA, Florida)

LM: Cercaria in skin

ND: Cercarial dermatitis due to *Gigantobilharzia huttoni*

TM: Skin penetration by cercaria in contaminated water

Leigh, W. H., 1955, The morphology of *Gigantobilharzia huttoni* (Leigh, 1953) an avian schistosome with marine dermatitis-producing larvae. *Journal of Parasitology*, **41**, 262–269.

Gigantobilharzia sturniae (Tanabe, 1948)

DH: Man; species of bird including *Motacilla grandis* (Japanese wagtail), *Passer montanus* (tree sparrow) and *Sturnia cinerazea* (starling)

IH: *Segmentina nitidella* (snail)

GD: Asia (Japan)

LM: Cercaria in skin

ND: Cercarial dermatitis due to *Gigantobilharzia sturniae*

TM: Skin penetration by cercaria in contaminated water

Oshima, T., Saito, K., Kitaguchi, T., Okuda, N., Kanazawa, M., Kanayama, A. and Masuda, C., 1988, Survey on the cercarial dermatitis appeared in Midori-Ku, Yokohama City, *Japanese Journal of Parasitology*, **37**, 97.

Heterobilharzia americana Price, 1929

DH: Man; many domesticated and wild species of mammal

IH: *Pseudosuccinea columella* (natural) and *Fossaria* sp. and *Lymnaea* sp. (experimental) (snails)

GD: The Americas (USA, Louisiana)

LM: Cercaria in skin

ND: Cercarial dermatitis due to *Heterobilharzia americana*

TM: Skin penetration by cercaria in contaminated water

Lee, H. F., 1962, Susceptibility of mammalian hosts to experimental infection with *Heterobilharzia americana*. *Journal of Parasitology*, **48**, 740-745.

Orientobilharzia turkestanica (Skrjabin, 1913) Srivastava, 1957

DH: Man; many domesticated and wild species of mammal

IH: Species of *Lymnaea* including *L. auriculata* (snails)

GD: Asia (China, Iran); helminth widely distributed in mammals in Asia

LM: Cercaria in skin

ND: Cercarial dermatitis due to *Orientobilharzia turkestanica*

TM: Skin penetration by cercaria in contaminated water

Sahba, G. H. and Malek, E. A., 1979, Dermatitis caused by cercariae of *Orientobilharzia turkestanicum* in the Caspian Sea area of Iran. *American Journal of Tropical Medicine and Hygiene*, **28**, 912-913.

Schistosomatium douthitti (Cort, 1914) Price 1931

DH: Man; wild species of rodent including *Microtus pennsylvanicus* (vole) and *Mus musculus* (mouse)

IH: Species of *Lymnaea* including *L. stagnalis*, also *Stagnicola emarginatus angulatus* (snails)

GD: The Americas (Canada, USA)

LM: Cercaria in skin

ND: Cercarial dermatitis due to *Schistosomatium douthitti*

TM: Skin penetration by cercaria in contaminated water

Cort, W. N., 1950, Studies on schistosome dermatitis. *American Journal of Hygiene*, **52**, 251–307.

Trichobilharzia brevis Basch, 1966

DH: Man; species of bird including *Anas platyrhynchos* (mallard)

IH: Species of *Lymnaea* including *L. rubiginosa* and *L. javanica*, also *Austropeplea ollula* (snails)

GD: Asia (Japan)

LM: Cercaria in skin

ND: Cercarial dermatitis due to *Trichobilharzia brevis*

TM: Skin penetration by cercaria in contaminated fresh water

Suzuki, N. and Kawanaka, M., 1980, *Trichobilharzia brevis* Basch, 1966, as a cause of an outbreak of cercarial dermatitis in Japan. *Japanese Journal of Parasitology*, **29**, 1–11.

Trichobilharzia ocellata (La Valette, 1855) Brumpt, 1931

DH: Man; many species of wildfowl (ducks)

IH: Species of *Lymnaea* and *Physa* including *L. stagnalis* and *P. integra* (snails)

GD: The Americas (USA); Africa (South Africa); Asia (India, Japan, Myanmar); Europe (France, Germany, Switzerland, UK); Oceania (New Zealand); helminth widely distributed in species of duck

LM: Cercaria in skin

ND: Cercarial dermatitis due to *Trichobilharzia ocellata*

TM: Skin penetration by cercaria in contaminated water

Eklu-Natey, D. T., Al-Khudri, M., Gauthey, D., Dubois, J. P., West, J., Vacher, C. and Huggel, H., 1985, Epidemiologie de la dermatite des baigneurs and morphologie de *Trichobilharzia* cf. *ocellata* dans le lac Leman. *Revue Suisse de Zoologie*, **92**, 939–953.

Trichobilharzia sp. (? *T.paoi*)

DH: Man; species of wildfowl

IH: *Radix cucunonica* (snail)

GD: Asia (China)

LM: Cercaria in skin

ND: Cercarial dermatitis due to *Trichobilharzia* sp.

TM: Skin penetration by cercaria in contaminated fresh water

Shao, G., 1988, Preliminary investigation on cercarial dermatitis in Ali Area of Xizang Autonomous Region, China. *Chinese Journal of Parasitology and Parasitic Diseases*, **6**, 169–170.

Trichobilharzia stagnicolae (Talbot, 1936)

DH: Man; species of wildfowl (experimentally in canary, duck, herring gull)

IH: Species of *Lymnaea* including *L. stagnalis* (snails)

GD: The Americas (USA)

LM: Cercaria in skin

ND: Cercarial dermatitis due to *Trichobilharzia stagnicolae*

TM: Skin penetration by cercaria in contaminated water

McMullen, D. B. and Beard, P. C., 1945, Studies on schistosome dermatitis. IX. The life cycles of three dermatitis producing schistosomes from birds and a discussion of the subfamily Bilharziellinae (Trematoda, Schistosomatidae). *American Journal of Hygiene*, **42**, 128–154.

CLINOSTOMATIDAE

Clinostomum complanatum (Rudolphi, 1814) Brown, 1899

DH: Man; species of fish-eating birds including *Ardea cinerea* (heron)

IH1:   Species of *Helisoma* including *H. antrosum* and *H. campanulatum* and of *Lymnaea* (snails)

IH2:   Many species of fish including *Carassius carassius* (carp), *Eupomotis gibbosus* and *Perca fluviatilis* (perch)

GD: Asia (Israel, Japan, Lebanon, Syrian Arab Republic); helminth widely distributed in animal hosts

LM: "... three adults ... on posterior wall of the pharynx of a human."

TM: Ingestion of metacercaria with infected raw or undercooked fish

Hirai, H., Ooiso, H., Kifune, T., Kiyota, T. and Sakaguchi, Y., 1987, *Clinostomum complanatum* infection in posterior wall of the pharynx of a human. *Japanese Journal of Parasitology*, **36**, 142–144.

CATHYCOTYLIDAE

Prohemistomum vivax (Sonsino, 1892) Azim, 1933

DH: MAN; domesticated cat and dog and *Milvus migrans aegyptiacus* (Egyptian kite)

IH1: *Cleopatra bulimoides* and *Melanopsis praemorsa* (snails)

IH2: Species of fish of the genera *Clarias, Mugil* and *Tilapia*

GD: Africa (Egypt)

LM: "... one case of a human infection ... More than 2000 adults recovered from the intestine ..." (Ulmer, 1975, In *Diseases Transmitted from Animals to Man* p. 646)

TM: Ingestion of metacercaria with infected raw, salted or undercooked fish

Nasr, M., 1941, The occurrence of *Prohemistomum vivax* (Sonsino, 1892) Azim, 1933. Infection in man, with a redescription of the parasite. *Laboratory Medical Progress*, **2**, 135–149.

DIPLOSTOMATIDAE

Alaria americana Hall and Wigdor, 1918

DH: Species of carnivorous mammal including domesticated cat and dog and *Vulpes pennsylvanica* (fox)

IH1: Possibly *Planorbis* spp. (snails)

IH2: *Rana* spp (frog, tadpole stage)

PH: Man; species of frog and snake

GD: The Americas (USA, Canada)

LM: Mesocercaria found in eye, lung, liver, heart, kidney, pancreas, stomach, spleen, lymph nodes, adipose tissue, brain and spinal cord

TM: Ingestion of mesocercaria with infected raw or undercooked frogs' legs or snakes; possibly by accidental transportation to eye whilst preparing food.

Freeman, R. S., Stuart, P. F., Cullen, J. B., Ritchie, A. C., Mildon, A., Fernandes, B. J. and Bonin, R., 1976, Fatal human infection with mesocercariae of the trematode *Alaria americana*. *American Journal of Tropical Medicine and Hygiene*, **25**, 803–807.

Alaria marcianae (La Rue, 1917) Walton, 1950

DH: Species of carnivorous mammal including domesticated cat and *Vulpes pennsylvanica* (fox)

IH1: Possibly *Planorbis* spp. (snails)

IH2: Species of frog including *Rana clamitans*, *R.catesbeina* and *Hyla cinerea*; species of snake including *Agkistrodon piscivorus* (cottonmouth or water moccasin) and *Coluber constrictor* (racer)

PH: Man; species of mammal including *Didelphis virginiana* (opossum) and *Procyon lotor* (raccoon)

GD: The Americas (USA, Louisiana)

LM: Mesocercaria found in thigh region near the groin

TM: Ingestion of mesocercaria with infected raw or undercooked frog, snake, alligator, raccoon and opossum or possibly accidental ingestion during preparation of food

Shoop, W. L. and Corkum, K. C., 1981, Epidemiology of *Alaria marcianae* mesocercariae in Louisiana. *Journal of Parasitology*, **67**, 928–931.

Diplostomum spathaceum (Rudolphi, 1819) Olsson, 1876

DH: Species of piscivorous bird including *Larus argentatus* (herring gull) and *L. ridibundus* (black-headed gull)

IH1: *Lymnaea auricularia* (snail)

IH2: Man; species of freshwater fish including *Salmo gairdneri* (rainbow trout)

GD: Europe (Czechoslovakia); widely distributed in species of water bird

LM: Cercaria in skin

TM: Skin penetration by cercaria in contaminated water

Sevcova, M., Kolarova, L. and Gottwaldova, V., 1987, Cerkariova dermatida. *Ceskoslovenska Dermatologie*, **62**, 369–374.

Fibricola seoulensis Seo, Rim and Lee, 1964

DH: MAN; species of *Rattus* (rats)

IH1: *Hippeutis cantori* (snail)

IH2: *Rana nigromaculata* (frog, adult and tadpole stage)

PH: *Rhabdophis tigrinus* (snake)

GD: Asia (South Korea)

LM: "The eggs of *F. seoulensis* were observed [in stool samples] in 15 cases." Adult located in the alimentary tract.

TM: Ingestion of metacercaria with infected raw or undercooked frog or snake

Hong, S. T., Cho, T. K., Hong, S. J., Chai, J. Y., Lee, S. H. and Seo, B. S., 1984, Fifteen human cases of *Fibricola seoulensis* infection in Korea. *Korean Journal of Parasitology*, **22**, 61–65.

PARAMPHISTOMIDAE

Gastrodiscoides hominis (Lewis and McConnell, 1876) Leiper, 1913

DH: MAN; domesticated pig; *Macaca mulatta* (rhesus monkey), *Rattus brevicaudatus* (rat) and *Tragulus napu* (chevrotain)

IH: *Helicorbis coenosus* (planorbid snail, experimental)

A guide to human helminths

GD: Asia (India, Pakistan, Philippines, Vietnam); Europe (USSR)

LM: Adult found in the caecum and ascending colon

ND: Gastrodiscoidiasis due to *Gastrodiscoides hominis*

TM: Probably ingestion of metacercaria in contaminated food

Buckley, J. J. C., 1964, The problem of *Gastrodiscoides hominis* (Lewis and McConnell, 1876) Leiper, 1913. *Journal of Helminthology*, **38**, 1-6.

Watsonius watsoni (Conygham, 1904) Stiles and Goldberger, 1910

DH: MAN; species of non-human primate including *Cercopithecus callitrichus* (cercopithicid monkey), *Macacus cynomolgus* (crab-eating macaque) and *Papio sphinx* (baboon)

IH: Presumably species of snail

GD: Africa (Nigeria)

LM: Adult attached to mucosa of duodenum and jejunum (autopsy)

ND: Watsoniasis

TM: Presumably from ingestion of metacercaria in contaminated food

Pick, F., 1964, Informations nouvelles sur la distomatose a *Watsonius watsoni. Bulletin de Societe Pathologie Exotique*, **57**, 502-510.

FASCIOLIDAE

Fasciola gigantica Cobbold, 1855

DH: MAN; species of domesticated and wild ruminant including cattle and *Giraffa campelopardalis* (giraffe)

IH: *Lymnaea natalensis* and *Physopsis africana* (snails)

GD: Africa (Uganda, Zimbabwe); The Americas (USA, Hawaii); Asia (Iraq, Vietnam), Europe (USSR, Tashkent)

LM: Adult in liver and biliary system; larva undergoes tissue migration

ND: Fascioliasis due to *Fasciola gigantica*

TM: Ingestion of metacercaria with contaminated vegetation

Sadykov, V. M., 1988, Discovery of *Fasciola* in the deceased in the Samarkand Region. *Meditsinskaya Parazitologiya i Parazitarnye Bolezni*, **4**, 71–73.

Fasciola hepatica Linnaeus, 1758

DH: MAN; various species of domesticated and wild herbivorous mammal

IH: Species of *Lymnaea* including *L. truncatula* and *L. tomentosa* (snails)

GD: Helminth distributed worldwide in domesticated cattle and sheep in temperate climates

LM: Adult in liver and biliary system; larva undergoes tissue migration

ND: Fascioliasis due to *Fasciola hepatica*

TM: Ingestion of metacercaria with contaminated vegetation

Ripert, C., Tribouley, J., Luang Dinh Giap, G., Combe, A. and Laborde, M., 1987, Epidemiologie de la fasciolose humaine dans le Sud Ouest de la France. *Bulletin de la Societe Francaise de Parasitologie*, **5**, 227–230.

Fasciola indica Varma, 1953

DH: MAN; species of domesticated mammal

IH: *Lymnaea acuminata* (snail)

GD: Asia (India, Korea)

LM: Adult in biliary system; larva undergoes tissue migration

ND: Fascioliasis due to *Fasciola indica*

TM: Ingestion of metacercaria with contaminated vegetation

Hong, S. T., 1986, A human case of gallbladder fascioliasis in Korea. *Korean Journal of Parasitology*, **24**, 89–93.

Fasciolopsis buski (Lankester, 1857) Odhner, 1902

DH: MAN; domesticated dog and pig

IH: Species of snail including *Hippeutis cantori, Segmentina hemisphaerula* and *S. trochoides*

GD: Asia (Bangladesh, Cambodia, China, India, Laos, Malaysia, Taiwan, Thailand, Vietnam)

LM: Adult in small intestine; larva undergoes tissue migration

ND: Fasciolopsiasis due to *Fasciolopsis buski*

TM: Ingestion of metacercaria with contaminated vegetation including *Echiornia speciosa* (water hyacinth), *E. tuberosa* (water chestnut) and *Trapa natans* (water caltrops)

Chandra, S. S., 1976, A field study on the clinical aspect of *Fasciolopsis buski* infections in Uttar Pradesh. *Medical Journal of Armed Forces, India,* **32,** 181–189.

ECHINOSTOMATIDAE

Echinochasmus japonicus Tanabe, 1926

DH: MAN; domesticated cat and dog, *Nycticorax nycticorax* (night heron)

IH1: *Parafossarulus striatulus* (snail)

IH2: Species of freshwater fish including *Hemibarbus barbus* and *Plecoglossus altivelis* (perch), also *Rana rugosa* (frog, tadpole stage)

GD: Asia (China, Japan, Taiwan)

LM: Presumably adult in small intestine

TM: Ingestion of metacercaria with infected raw or undercooked freshwater fish

Lin, J. X., 1985, Epidemiological investigation and experimental infection of *Echinochasmus japonicus.* Journal of Parasitology and Parasitic Diseases, **3,** 89–91.

Echinochasmus jiufoensis Liang and Ke, 1988

DH: Man

IH1:   Unresolved

IH2:   Unresolved

GD: Asia (China)

LM: "... from the intestine of an autopsy of 6-month-old girl ..."

TM: Presumably ingestion of metacercaria

Liang, C. and Ke, X-L., 1988, *Echinochasmus jiufoensis* sp. nov. a human parasite from Guangzhon (Trematode: Echinostomatidae). *Acta Zootaxonomica Sinica*, **13**, 4–8.

Echinochasmus perfoliatus (von Ratz, 1908)

DH: MAN; domesticated cat, dog and pig

IH1:   *Bythnia leachi, Lymnaea stagnalis* and *Parafossarulus manchouricus* (snails)

IH2:   Species of freshwater fish including *Acheilognathus intermedius, Mogurnda obscura* and *Pelteobargus nudiceps*

GD: Asia (Japan, Taiwan); helminth widely distributed in Asia and Europe

LM: Small intestine

TM: Ingestion of metacercaria with raw or undercooked freshwater fish.

Tanabe, H., 1922, *Echinochasmus perfoliatus* (Ratz) found in Japan. *Journal of Okayama Medical Association* 287, 1–20.

Echinoparyphium recurvatum (Linstow, 1873) Luehe, 1909

DH: MAN; species of domesticated bird, *Strix* sp. (owl), experimentally in cat, dog and rat

IH1:   *Lymnaea swinhoei, L.ollula* and *Planorbis* sp. (snails)

IH2:   *Lymnaea swinhoei, L. ollula* and *Planorbis* sp. (snails); *Corbicula fluminea* (clam)

GD: Asia (Taiwan)

LM: Small intestine

TM: Ingestion of metacercaria with raw or undercooked mollusc

Lu, Sen-Chi, 1982, Echinostomiasis in Taiwan, *International Journal of Zoonoses*, **9**, 33–38.

Echinostoma cinetorchis Ando and Ozaki, 1923

DH: MAN; domesticated dog, rat and other species of mammal; domesticated fowl and species of bird

IH1:   *Segmentina nitidella* (snail)

IH2:   *Planorbis compressus japonicus, Segmentina nitidella* and *Viviparus malleatus* (snails); *Rana japonica, R. nigromaculata* and *R. rugosa* (frogs, adult and tadpole)

GD: Asia (Japan, Korea, Taiwan)

LM: Small intestine; "... eggs found in the stools ..."

ND: Echinostomiasis due to *Echinostoma cinetorchis*

TM: Ingestion of metacercaria with raw or undercooked snails

Ryang, Y. S., Ahn, Y. K., Kim, W. T., Shin, K. C., Lee, K. W. and Kim, T. S., 1986, Two cases of human infection by *Echinostoma cinetorchis*, *Korean Journal of Parasitology*, **24**, 71–76.

Echinostoma echinatum (Zeder, 1803)

DH: MAN; experimentally in duck, mouse, pigeon and rat

IH1:   *Gyraulus convexiusculus* and *Anisus (Gyraulus) sarasinorum* (snails)

IH2:   Species of freshwater mollusc including *Corbicula lindoensis* (clam) and *Viviparus javanicus* (snail)

GD: Asia (Indonesia)

LM: Small intestine

ND: Echinostomiasis due to *Echinostoma lindoense*

TM: Ingestion of metacercaria with raw or undercooked freshwater mollusc

Huffman, J. E. and Fried, B., 1990, *Echinostoma* and Echinostomiasis, *Advances in Parasitology*, **29**, 215–269.

Echinostoma hortense Asada, 1926

DH: MAN; rat and other species of rodents

IH1:   *Lymnaea japonica, L. ollula* and *L. pervia* (snails)

IH2:   *Rana caresbiana, R. nigromaculata* and *R. ongosa* (frogs, adult and tadpole), also species of freshwater fish including *Misgurnus anguilli-caudatus* (loach)

GD: Asia (China, Japan, Korea)

LM: Small intestine

ND: Echinostomiasis due to *Echinostoma hortense*

TM: Ingestion of metacercaria with raw or undercooked frogs or freshwater fish

Lee, S. K., Chung, N. S., Ko, I. H. and Ko, H. I., 1986, Two cases of natural human infection by *Echinostoma hortense*. *Korean Journal of Parasitology*, **24**, 77–81.

Echinostoma ilocanum (Garrison, 1908) Odhner, 1911

DH: MAN; domesticated cat and dog

IH1:   *Gyraulus convexiusculus, G. prashadi* and *Hippeutis umbilicalis* (snails)

IH2:   *G. prashadi, Pila ampullacea, P. luzonica* and *Vivipara burranghina* (snails)

GD: Asia (China; Indonesia, Celebes, Java; Malaysia; Philippines)

LM: Small intestine

ND: Echinostomiasis due to *Echinostoma ilocanum*

TM: Ingestion of metacercaria with raw or undercooked freshwater molluscs

Kumar, V., 1987, Zoonotic trematodiasis in south-east and far-east Asian countries. In *Helminth Zoonoses* edited by S. Geert, V. Kumar and J. Brandt. (Dordrecht, Boston, Lancaster: Martinus Nijhoff Publishers) pp. 106–117.

Echinostoma macrorchis Ando and Ozaki, 1923

DH: MAN: *Rattus norvegicus* and *R. rattus* (rats), *Capella gallinago* (snipe)

IH1: *Parafossarulus compressus japonicus* and *Segmentina nitidella* (snails)

IH2: *Parafossarulus compressus japonicus, P. manchouricus, Segmentina nitidella* and *Viviparus malleatus* (snails)

GD: Asia (Japan)

LM: Small intestine

ND: Echinostomiasis due to *Echinostoma macrorchis*

TM: Ingestion of metacercaria with raw or undercooked snails

Majima, M., 1927, On *Echinostoma macrorchis* found in man, *Kumamoto Igakkai Zasshi* 2552, 2260. (Original not seen, quoted by Rim, 1982. CRC *Parasitic Zoonoses*, III. pp. 53–69).

Echinostoma malayanum Leiper, 1911

DH: MAN; domesticated pig, rat and *Suncus mucrinus* (house shrew)

IH1: *Lymnaea luteola* (snail)

IH2: *Bellamya ingallsiana, Gyraulus convexiusculus, Indoplanorbis exustus, Lymnaea luteola* and *Pila scutata* (snails) also *Barbus stigma* (barbel)

GD: Asia (Indonesia, Malaysia, Singapore, Thailand)

LM: Small intestine

ND: Echinostomiasis due to *Echinostoma malayanum*

TM: Ingestion of metacercaria with raw or undercooked freshwater snails or fish

Lie-Kian Joe and Virik, H. K. 1963, Human infection with *Echinostoma malayanum* Leiper, 1911 (Trematoda. Echinostomidae). *Journal of Tropical Medicine and Hygiene,* **66,** 77–82.

Echinostoma revolutum (Froelich, 1802) Looss, 1899

DH: MAN; *Ondatra zibethicus* (muskrat), species of domesticated bird, dog and rat (experimental)

IH1: *Helisoma trivolvis* and *Stagnicola palustris* (snails)

IH2: Species of mollusc including *Corbicula fluminea* (clam), *Helisoma trivolvis, Stagnicola palustris* and *Vivipara vivipara* (snails)

GD: Asia (Indonesia, Taiwan)

LM: Small intestine

ND: Echinostomiasis due to *Echinostoma revolutum*

TM: Ingestion of metacercaria with raw or undercooked freshwater molluscs

Lu, S-C., 1982, Echinostomiasis in Taiwan. *International Journal of Zoonoses,* **9,** 33–38.

Episthmium caninum (Verma, 1935) Yamaguti, 1958

DH: MAN; domesticated dog

IH1: Presumably species of snail

IH2: Unresolved

GD: Asia (Thailand)

LM: "... has been recovered, on one occasion from the stools of a patient ... in Bangkok."

TM: Presumably ingestion of metacercaria

CIOMS/WHO, 1987. *International Nomenclature of Diseases.* II. *Infectious Diseases.* Part 4: Parasitic Diseases. Geneva: W.H.O., p. 41

Euparyphium melis (Schrank, 1788)

DH: MAN

IH1:   Presumably species of snail

IH2:   Unresolved

GD: Asia (China); Europe (Romania)

LM: Small intestine

TM: Presumably ingestion of metacercaria

Hsu, H. F., 1940, *Euparyphium jassyense* Leon and Ciurea(= *E.melis* Schrank) found at autopsy of a Chinese. *Chinese Medical Journal*, **58**, 552–558.

Himasthala muehlensi Vogel, 1933

DH: MAN

IH1:   Presumably species of snail

IH2:   Presumably *Venus mercenaria* (clam)

GD: The Americas (Colombia; USA?)

Loan Receipt

Liverpool John Moores University
Learning and Information Services

Borrower ID: 21111093276129

Loan Date: 23/01/2009
Loan Time: 5:13 pm

The war within us :
31111008799379
Due Date: 13/02/2009 23:59

A guide to human helminths /
31111004553887
Due Date: 30/01/2009 23:59

Basic clinical parasitology /
31111006269946
Due Date: 13/02/2009 23:59

Handbook of medical parasitology /
31111003839915
Due Date: 13/02/2009 23:59

Medical parasitology /
31111006243339
Due Date: 13/02/2009 23:59

Please keep your receipt
in case of dispute

LM: Presumably small intestine; "... five specimens ... were obtained from a German patient, who had lived for 6 years in Colombia, but believed he acquired the infection from consuming several raw clams (*Venus mercenaria*) in New York City."

TM: Presumably ingestion of metacercaria

Rim, H.-J., 1982, Echinostomiasis. In *C.R.C. Handbook Series in Zoonoses.* Section C. *Parasitic Zoonoses* III, edited by G. V. Hillyer and C. E. Hopla, (Boca Raton, Florida: CRC Press, Inc.), pp. 53–69.

Hypoderaeum conoideum (Bloch, 1782) Dietz, 1908

DH: MAN; species of domesticated and wild anseriform and galliform bird

IH1: *Lymnaea stagnalis* and *Planorbis corneus* (snails)

IH2: Snails and tadpoles in Thailand

GD: Asia (Taiwan, Thailand)

LM: Small intestine

TM: Ingestion of metacercaria with raw or undercooked snail

Yokogawa, M., Harinasuta, C. and Charoenlap, P., 1965, *Hypoderaeum conoideum* (Bloch, 1782) Dietz, 1909, a common intestinal fluke in man in Northeast Thailand. *Japanese Journal of Parasitology*, **14**, 148–153.

PSILOSTOMATIDAE

Psilorchis hominis Kifune and Takao, 1973

DH: Man; possibly species of bird

IH1: Unresolved

IH2: Unresolved; possibly species of freshwater fish or mollusc

GD: Asia (Japan)

LM: Presumably in small intestine

TM: Presumably ingestion of metacercaria with raw or undercooked second intermediate host

Kifune, T. and Takao, Y., 1973, Description of *Psilorchis hominis* sp. nov. from man (Trematoda: Echinostomatoidea: Psilostomidae). *Japanese Journal of Parasitology*, **22,** 111–115.

LECITHODENDRIIDAE

Phaneropsolus bonnei (Lie-Kian Joe, 1951)

DH: MAN; *Macaca irus* (crab-eating macaque), *M. mulatta* (rhesus monkey) and *Nycticebus coucang* (slow loris)

IH1:   Unresolved

IH2:   Unresolved

GD: Asia (Thailand)

LM: Small intestine

TM: Presumably ingestion of metacercaria

Manning, G. S. and Viyanant, V., 1970, Report of *Phaneropsolus bonnei* Lie-Kian Joe 1951. (Trematoda; Lecithodendriidae) from humans in northeastern Thailand. *Southeast Asian Journal of Tropical Medicine and Public Health*, **1**, 427–428.

Prosthodendrium molenkampi (Lie-Kian Joe, 1951)

DH: MAN; rat, and *Scotophilus kuhli* and *Taphozous melanopogon* (bats)

IH1:   Unresolved

IH2:   Unresolved

GD: Asia (Indonesia)

LM: "... recovered from autopsies ...", presumably in small intestine

TM: Unresolved

Manning, G. S., Viyanant, V., Lertprasert, P., Watanasirmkit, K. and Chetty, C., 1970, Three new human trematodes from Thailand. *Southeast Asian Journal of Tropical Medicine and Public Health*, **1**, 560.

PLAGIORCHIIDAE

Plagiorchis harinasutai Radomyos, Bunnag and Harinasuta, 1989

DH: MAN

IH1: Unresolved

IH2: Unresolved

GD: Asia (Thailand)

LM: Small intestine

TM: Presumably ingestion of metacercaria

Radomyos, P., Bunnag, D. and Harinasuta, T., 1989, A new intestinal fluke *Plagiorchis harinasutai* n.sp. *Southeast Asian Journal of Tropical Medicine and Public Health*, **20**, 101–107.

Plagiorchis javensis Sandground, 1940

DH: MAN

IH1: Unresolved

IH2: Unresolved

GD: Asia (Indonesia)

LM: Small intestine

TM: Presumably ingestion of metacercaria

Kwo En Hoa and Lie, K. J., 1953. Occurrence in man in Indonesia of trematodes commonly found in animals. *Journal of Indonesian Medical Association*, **3**, 131–136.

Plagiorchis muris Tanabe, 1922

DH: MAN; domesticated dog and sheep, rat and various species of bird

IH1: *Lymnaea pervia* and *L. japonica* (snails)

IH2:   *Chironomus dorsalis* (midge) and *Lymnaea emerginata angulata* (snail)

GD: Asia (Japan)

LM: Small intestine

TM: Presumably ingestion of metacercaria with second intermediate host

Asada, J. L., Otagaki, H., Morita, D., Takeuchi, T., Sakai, Y., Konishi, T. and Okahashi, K., 1962; A case report on the human infection with *Plagiorchis muris* Tanabe, 1922. *Japanese Journal of Parasitology*, **11**, 512–516.

Plagiorchis philippinensis Sandground, 1940

DH: MAN

IH1:   Unresolved

IH2:   Species of insect

GD: Asia (Philippines)

LM: Small intestine

TM: Presumably ingestion of metacercaria

Africa, C. M. and Garcia, E. Y., 1937, *Plagiorchis* sp. new trematode parasite of the human intestine. *Papers on Helminthology*, 30 year Jubileum K. J. Skrjabin, Moscow, 9–10.

CATHAEMASIIDAE

Cathaemasia cabrerai Juneco and Monzon, 1984

DH: MAN; possibly species of bird

IH1:   Unresolved

IH2:   Unresolved

GD: Asia (Philippines)

LM: "... stool examination ... showed the presence of eggs ... 32 worms were recovered."

TM: Presumably ingestion of metacercaria

Jueco, N. L. and Monzon, R. B., 1984, *Cathaemasia cabrerai* Sp.N. (Trematoda: Cathaemasiidae) a new parasite of man in the Philippines. *Southeast Asian Journal of Tropical Medicine and Public Health*, **15**, 427–429.

PHILOPHTHALMIDAE

Philophthalmus lacrymosus Braun, 1902

DH: Man; *Larus maculipennis* (seagull), *Casmerodius albus egretta* (egret) and other species of bird

IH: Unresolved

GD: Europe (Yugoslavia)

LM: Eye (conjunctival sac)

TM: Unresolved; possibly direct contact with cercaria in water

Markovich, A., 1939, Der erste Fall von Philophthalmose beim Menschen. *Archiv fur Opthalmologie*, **140**, 515–526.

Philophthalmus sp.

DH: Man; species of aquatic bird

IH: Unresolved

GD: Asia (Sri Lanka)

LM: Conjunctiva; "... patient ... complained of irritation in ... right eye ... the worm emerged."

TM: Unresolved; possibly cercarial invasion while bathing

Dissanaike, A. S. and Bilimoria, D. P., 1958, On an infection of a human eye with *Philophthalmus* sp. in Ceylon. *Journal of Helminthology*, **32**, 115–118.

DICROCOELIIDAE

Dicrocoelium dendriticum (Rudolphi, 1819) Looss, 1899

DH: MAN; many species of mammal including sheep and other domesticated ruminant herbivores

IH1: Many species of terrestrial snail including *Helix vulgaris*, *Cochlicopha lubrica* and *Lacinaria varnensis*

IH2: Seventeen species of ant including *Formica fusca* and *Proformica nasuta*

GD: Helminth widely distributed, recorded occasionally from humans worldwide

LM: Biliary system

ND: Dicrocoeliasis due to *Dicrocoelium dendriticum*

TM: Accidental ingestion of metacercaria in ant or from contaminated vegetation

Drabick, J. J., Brown, S. L., Vick, R. G., Sandman, B. M. and Neafie, R. C., 1988, Dicroceliasis (lancet fluke disease) in an HIV seropositive man. *Journal of the American Medical Association*, **259**, 567–568.

Dicrocoelium hospes Looss, 1907

DH: MAN; species of domesticated and wild herbivorous mammal

IH1: Species of *Achatina* and *Limicolaria* (snails)

IH2: Species of *Crematogaster* and *Dorylus* (ants)

GD: Africa (Ethiopia, Ghana*, Kenya, Sierra Leone)

LM: Biliary system

ND: Dicrocoeliasis due to *Dicrocoelium hospes*

TM: Accidental ingestion of metacercaria in ant

Chunge, R. N. and Desai, M., 1989, Short communication: A human infection with *Dicrocoelium* in Kenya. *East African Medical Journal*, **66**, 551–552.

* some cases may be spurious infection

Eurytrema pancreaticum (Janson, 1889) Looss, 1907

DH: MAN; domesticated buffalo, camel, cattle, goat and sheep and *Macaca syrichta fascicularis* (monkey)

IH1: *Bradybaena similaris* (terrestrial snail)

IH2: *Conocephalus maculatus* (grasshopper)

GD: Asia (China, Japan); helminth widely distributed in Southeast Asia and South America.

LM: Pancreatic duct

TM: Presumably from accidental ingestion of metacercaria in grasshopper

Ishii, Y., Koga, M., Fujino, T., Higo, H., Ishibashi, J., Oka, K. and Saito, S., 1983, Human infection with the pancreas liver fluke, *Eurytrema pancreaticum. American Journal of Tropical Medicine and Hygiene*, **32**, 1019-1022

PARAGONIMIDAE

Paragonimus africanus Voelker and Vogel, 1965

DH: MAN; domesticated dog, *Crossarchus obscurus* (mongoose) and *Viverra civetta* (African civet cat)

IH1: Presumably species of snail

IH2: *Sudanonautes africanus* and *S. pelli* (crabs)

GD: Africa (Cameroon, Nigeria)

LM: Lungs

ND: Paragonimiasis due to *Paragonimus africanus*

TM: Ingestion of metacercaria with raw or undercooked crab

Voelker, J. and Vogel, H., 1985, Zwei neue *Paragonimus*-Arten aus West-Africa: *Paragonimus africanus* and *Paragonimus uterobilateralis* (Troglotrematidae: Trematoda). *Tropenmedezin Parasitologie*, **16**, 125-148.

Paragonimus bangkokensis

DH: Man

IH1: Presumably species of snail

IH2: Presumably species of crab or crayfish

GD: Europe (USSR)

LM: Unresolved

TM: Presumably ingestion of metacercaria

Kurochkin, Y. V., 1987, [Trematodes of the Fauna of SSSR, Paragonimids] "Nauka'', Moscow, 152 pp.

Paragonimus caliensis Little, 1968

DH: MAN; *Didelphis marsupialis* and *Philander opossum* (opossums)

IH1: *Aroapyrgus columbiensis* (snail)

IH2: Species of *Strengeria* (river crab)

GD: The Americas (Colombia)

LM: Presumably lungs

ND: Paragonimiasis due to *Paragonimus caliensis*

TM: Presumably ingestion of metacercaria with raw or undercooked crab

Kurochkin, Y. V. and Sukhanova, G. I., 1978, Species composition of the genus *Paragonimus*. Meditsinskaya Parazitologiyai Parazitarnye Bolezni, **47**, 36–39.

Paragonimus heterotremus Chen and Hsia, 1964

DH: MAN; domesticated cat and dog, and rat

IH1: *Tricula gregoriana* (snail)

IH2:   *Parathelphusa dugasti* and *Potamon smithianum* (crabs)

GD: Asia (China, Laos, Thailand)

LM: Lungs

ND: Paragonimiasis due to *Paragonimus heterotremus*

TM: Presumably ingestion of metacercaria with raw or undercooked second intermediate host

Miyazaki, I. and Fontan, R., 1970, Mature *Paragonimus heterotremus* found in man in Laos. *Japanese Journal of Parasitology*, **19**, 109–113.

Paragonimus hueit'ungensis Chung, Hsu, Ho, Kao, Shaw, Ch'iu, Pi, Liu, Ouyang, Shen, Yi and Yao, 1975

DH: Man; domesticated cat and dog, and rat (experimental)

IH1:   *Tricula cristella* (snail)

IH2:   *Isolapotamon papilonaceus, I. sinense, Sinopotamon denticulatum* and *S. joshueiense* (crabs)

GD: Asia (China)

LM: "Migratory subcutaneous nodules …"

ND: Paragonimiasis due to *Paragonimus hueit'ungensis*

TM: Ingestion of metacercaria with raw or undercooked crab

Chung, H. L., Hsu, C. P., Ho, L. Y., Kao, P. C., Lan, S. and Chiu, F. H., 1977, Studies on a new pathogenic lung fluke *Paragonimus hueit' ungensis* sp. nov. *Chinese Medical Journal*, **3**, 374–394.

Paragonimus kellicotti Ward, 1908

DH: MAN; domesticated cat, dog and pig, *Didelphys marsupialis* (opossum), *Felis rufa, Mustela vison* (mink) and *Procyon lotor* (raccoon)

IH1:   *Pomatiopsis lapidaria* (snail)

IH2:   Species of *Cambarus* (crayfish)

GD: The Americas (Canada)

LM: Lungs

ND: Paragonimiasis due to *Paragonimus kellicotti*

TM: Ingestion of metacercaria with raw or undercooked crayfish.

Bleland, J. E., Boone, J., Donevan, R. E. and Mankiewicz, E., 1969, Paragonimiasis (the lung fluke). Report of four cases. *American Review of Respiratory Diseases*, **99**, 261–271.

Paragonimus mexicanus Miyazaki and Ishii, 1968

DH: MAN; domesticated cat and dog, *Didelphis marsupialis* (opossum), *Nasua nasua* (coati) and *Procyon lotor* (raccoon)

IH1:   *Araopyrgus costaricensis* (snail)

IH2:   *Potamocarcinus magnus, Pseudothelphusa dilata* and *Ptycophallus* sp. (crabs)

GD: The Americas (Mexico, possibly also in Costa Rica, Guatemala and Panama)

LM: "… lung tissue excised from a Mexican male patient of 35 years old."

ND: Paragonimiasis due to *Paragonimus mexicanus*

TM: Ingestion of metacercaria with raw or undercooked crab

Miyazaki, I. and Ishii, Y., 1968, Studies on the Mexican lung flukes, with special reference to a description of *Paragonimus mexicanus* sp. nov., (Trematoda: Troglotrematidae). *Japanese Journal of Parasitology*, **17**, 445–453.

Paragonimus miyazakii Kamo, Nishida, Hatsushika and Tomimura, 1961

DH: MAN; domesticated cat and dog, species of wild carnivore including *Martes martes* (pine martin) and *Meles meles* (badger)

IH1:   *Bythinella nipponica akiyoshiensis, B.n.nipponica* and *Saganda* sp. (snails)

IH2: *Potamon (Geothelphusa) dehaani* (crab)

GD: Asia (Japan)

LM: Lungs and abdomen

ND: Paragonimiasis due to *Paragonimus miyazakii*

TM: Ingestion of metacercaria with raw or undercooked crab.

Yokogawa, M., Araki, K., Saito, K., Momose, T., Kimura, M., Suzuki, S., Chiba, N., Kitsumi, H. and Minai, M., 1974, *Paragonimus miyazakii* infections in man first found in Kamo district, Japan - especially on the methods of immuno-serodiagnosis for paragonimiasis. *Japanese Journal of Parasitology*, **23**, 167–179.

Paragonimus ohirai Miyazaki, 1939

DH: MAN; rat (experimental)

IH1: Possibly *Angustassiminea parasitologica* (snail)

IH2: *Sesarma dehaani* (crab)

GD: Asia (Japan)

LM: Presumably lungs

ND: Paragonimiasis due to *Paragonimus ohirai*

TM: Presumably ingestion of metacercaria

Yamaguchi, T., Sakurada, T. and Minami, Y., 1988, A case of *Paragonimus ohirai* infection. In: Proceedings of the Regional Meetings of the Japanese Society of Parasitology (No. 2). *Japanese Journal of Parasitology*, **37**, 82.

Paragonimus philippinensis Ito, Yokogawa, Araki and Kobayashi, 1978

DH: MAN; domesticated dog and rat (experimental)

IH1: *Antemelenia asperta* and *A. dactylus* (snails)

IH2: *Parathelphusa (Barythelphusa) grospoides* and *Sundathelphusa philipina* (crabs)

GD: Asia (Philippines)

LM: Lungs

ND: Paragonimiasis due to *Paragonimus philippinensis*

TM: Ingestion of metacercaria with raw or undercooked crab

Ito, J., Yokogawa, M., Araki, K. and Kobayashi, M., 1979, Further observations on the morphology of adult lung fluke, *Paragonimus philippinensis* Ito, Yokogawa, Araki and Kobayashi, 1978. *Japanese Journal of Parasitology*, **28**, 253–259.

Paragonimus pulmonalis (Baelz, 1883) Miyazaki, 1978

DH: MAN; domesticated cat and dog

IH1: *Semisulcospira libertina* and *Brotia costula episcopalis* (snails)

IH2: Species of crustacean including *Cambaroides similis*, *Eriochier japonicus* (crab), *Palaemon nipponensis* (shrimp) and *Procambarus clarkii* (crayfish)

PH: *Sus scrofa leucomystax* (Japanese wild boar)

GD: Asia (Japan, Korea, Taiwan)

LM: Lungs

ND: Paragonimiasis due to *Paragonimus pulmonalis*

TM: Ingestion of metacercarcia with raw or undercooked second inter-mediate host or larval form in paratenic host

Miyazaki, I., 1978, Two types of lung fluke which has been called *Paragonimus westermani* (Kerbert, 1878). *Medical Bulletin Fukuoka University*, **5**, 251–263.

Paragonimus sadoensis Miyazaki, Kawashima, Hamajina and Otsuru, 1968

DH: Man; rat (experimental)

IH1: Possibly *Oncomelania minima* (snail)

IH2:   *Potamon dehaani* (crab)

GD: Asia (Japan)

LM: Lungs

TM: Presumably ingestion of metacercaria with raw or undercooked crab

Kurochkin, Y. V. and Sukharova, G. I., 1978, The species composition of the genus *Paragonimus* and the causative agents of paragonimiasis in humans. *Meditinskia Parasitologia e Parazitarnia Bolesni*, **47**, 36–39.

Paragonimus skrjabini Chen, 1960

S: *P. szechuanensis*

DH: MAN; domesticated cat and dog, *Paguma larvata* (masked palm civet)

IH1:   *Assiminea lutea* and *Tricula gregoriana* (snails)

IH2:   *Sinopotamon denticulatum* and *S. yaanense* (crabs)

GD: Asia (China)

LM: Lungs, subcutaneous and cerebral tissue

ND: Paragonimiasis due to *Paragonimus skrjabini*

TM: Ingestion of metacercaria with raw or undercooked crab

Wang, X., Liu, Y., Wang, Q., Zhan, Q., Yu, M. and Yu, D., 1985, Clinical analysis of 119 cases of *Paragonimiasis szchuanensis*. *Journal of Parasitology and Parasitic Diseases*, **3**, 5–8.

Paragonimus uterobilateralis Voelker and Vogel, 1965

DH: MAN; species of non-human primate including *Mandrillus leucophaeus* (drill) and *Periodicitus potto* (potto), domesticated dog, species of wild carnivore including *Atilax paludinosus* (swamp mongoose), *Crossarchus obscurus* (long nosed mongoose) and *Viverra civetta* (African civet cat)

IH1:   Probably *Afropomus balanoides* and *Potadoma sanctipauli* (snails)

IH2:   *Liberonautes latidactylus, Sudanonautes africanus* and *S. aubryi* (crabs)

GD: Africa (Cameroon, Liberia, Nigeria)

LM: Lungs

ND: Paragonimiasis due to *Paragonimus uterobilateralis*

TM: Ingestion of metacercaria with raw or undercooked crab

Sachs, R., 1987, Occurrence of human lung fluke infection in an endemic area in Liberia. In *Helminth Zoonoses* edited by S. Geerts, V. Kumar and J. Brandt (Dordrecht, Boston, Lancaster: Martinus Nijhoff Publishers), pp. 132–136.

Paragonimus westermani (Kerbert, 1878) Brown, 1899

DH: MAN; domesticated cat, dog and pig; species of wild carnivore including *Canis lupus* (wolf), *Herpestes urva* (crab-eating mongoose) and *Viverra zibetha ashtoni* (civet cat)

IH1:   *Brotia costula episcopalis* and *Semisulcospira libertina* (snails)

IH2:   *Eriocheir sinensis, E. japonicus, Potamon denticulatus* and *P. smithianus* (crabs) also *Cambaroides similis* (crayfish)

PH: *Sus scrofa leucomystax* (Japanese wild boar)

GD: Asia (China, India, Indonesia, Japan, Korea, Malaysia, Myanmar, Nepal, New Guinea, Sri Lanka, Taiwan, Thailand); Europe (USSR)

LM: Lungs, cerebral subcutaneous tissue and other parenteral sites

ND: Paragonimiasis due to *Paragonimus westermani*

TM: Ingestion of metacercaria with raw, pickled or undercooked crab or crayfish

Yokogawa, M., 1965, *Paragonimus* and paragonimiasis. *Advances in Parasitology*, **3**, 99–158.

Paragonimus* sp.

DH: MAN

IH1: Unresolved

IH2: Unresolved

GD: The Americas (Peru)

LM: "... demonstrated two lung flukes [with eggs] ... from a worm cyst in the right lung of a 36-year-old Peruvian male."

TM: Presumably ingestion of metacercaria with raw or undercooked second intermediate host

Miyazaki, I., Arellano, C. and Grados, O., 1972, The first demonstration of the lungfluke, *Paragonimus* from man in Peru. *Japanese Journal of Parasitology*, **21**, 168-172.

ACHILLURBAINIIDAE

Achillurbainia nouveli Dollfus, 1939

DH: MAN; *Panthera pardus* (Malay panther)

IH1: Unresolved

IH2: *Paratelphusa rugosa* (crab) in Sri Lanka

GD: Asia (China)

LM: Retroauricular nodule

TM: Presumably ingestion of metacercaria with raw or undercooked crab

Kannangara, D. W. W., 1971, *Paratelphusa rugosa* as the second intermediate host of *Achillurbainia* a trematode transmissible to man. *Journal of Parasitology*, **57**, 683-684

---

* Not *Paragonimus amazonicus*, see Miyazaki *et al.*, 1973, *Jap. J. Parasit.*, **22**, 48-54.

Achillurbainia recondita Travassos, 1942

DH: Man; *Didelphis marsupialis* (opossum) and *Rattus muelleri* (rat)

IH1:   Unresolved

IH2:   Unresolved

GD: The Americas (Honduras; USA, Louisiana; Brazil)

LM: Omentum and other peritoneal surfaces.

TM: Presumably ingestion of metacercaria

Beaver, P. C., Little, M. D., Tucker, C. F. and Reed, R. J., 1977, Mesocercaria in the skin of man in Louisiana. *American Journal of Tropical Medicine and Hygiene*, **26**, 422–426.

Poikilorchis congolensis Fain and Vandepitte, 1957

DH: Man

IH: Unresolved

GD: Africa (Nigeria)

LM: "… operculated eggs in pus from mastoid abscess … No adult worm was recovered … the exact identification … remains uncertain."

TM: Presumably ingestion of infective stage

Oyediran, A. B. O. O., Fajemisin, A. A., Abioye, A. A., Lagundoye, S. B. and Olubile, A. O. B., 1975, Infection of the mastoid bone with a *Paragonimus*-like trematode. *American Journal of Tropical Medicine and Hygiene*, **24**, 268–273.

NANOPHYETIDAE

Nanophyetus salmincola salmincola (Chapin, 1926) Chapin, 1927

DH: MAN; domesticated cat and dog, species of wild carnivorous mammal including *Mustela vison* (mink), *Procyon lotor* (raccoon), *Spilogale putarius* (spotted skunk) and *Vulpes fulva* (fox) and species of piscivorous bird including *Ardea herodias* (heron)

IH1:   *Goniobasis plicifera silicula* and *Oxytrema silicula* (snails)

IH2: Species of salmonid fish including *Oncorhynchus kisutch, O. mykiss* and *O. tschamytscha*

GD: The Americas (USA)

LM: Small intestine; "... cases of stool-proven nanophyetiasis ..."

ND: Nanophyetiasis due to *Nanophyetus salmincola*

TM: Ingestion of metacercaria in raw, smoked or undercooked fish

Eastburn, R. L., Fritsche, T. R. and Terhune, C. A., 1987, Human intestinal infection with *Nanophyetus salmincola* from salmonid fishes. *American Journal of Tropical Medicine and Hygiene*, **36**, 586–591.

Nanophyetus salmincola schikhobalowi Skrjabin and Podjapolshaja, 1931

DH: Man; domesticated cat and dog, species of wild carnivorous mammal including *Meles meles* (badger), *Mustela vison* (mink) and *Vulpes vulpes* (red fox)

IH1: *Semisulcospira cancellata* and *S. laevigata* (snails)

IH2: Species of fish including *Coregonus ussuriensis* (whitefish), *Cyprinus carpo* (carp), *Phoxinus phoxinus* (minnow) and *Savelinus malma* (Dolly Varden)

GD: Europe (USSR, Siberia)

LM: Small intestine

ND: Nanophyetiasis due to *Nanophyetus salmincola schikhobalowi*

TM: Ingestion of metacercaria in infected raw, smoked or undercooked fish

Millemann, R. E. and Knapp, S. E., 1970, Biology of *Nanophyetus salmincola* and "Salmon Poisoning" Disease. *Advances in Parasitology*, **8**, 1–41.

OPISTHORCHIDAE

Metorchis albidus (Braun, 1893) Looss, 1899

DH: Man; domesticated cat and dog, various species of piscivorous mammal

IH1: Unresolved

IH2: Species of fish including *Carassius carassius* (crucian carp) and *Gobio gobio* (gudgeon)

GD: The Americas (USA, Alaska); Europe (France, USSR)

LM: Presumably in the biliary system

TM: Ingestion of metacercaria with raw or undercooked fish

Sidorov, E. G. and Belyakova, 1972, Natural nidus of *Metorchis* and the biology of the agent. In: Contributions to the natural nidality of diseases. *Acad. Sci. Kazakh*, **5**, 133–150.

Metorchis conjunctus (Cobbold, 1864) Looss, 1899

DH: MAN; domesticated cat and dog, *Mustela vison* (mink), *Procyon lotor* (raccoon) and *Vulpes vulpes* (red fox)

IH1: *Amnicola limosa porata* (snail)

IH2: *Catostomus commersonii* (common sucker)

GD: The Americas (Canada, Greenland)

LM: Presumably in the biliary system. (Eggs have been recovered from stools)

TM: Ingestion of metacercaria with infected raw or undercooked fish

Babbott, F. L., Frye, W. W. and Gordon, J. E., 1961, Intestinal parasites of man in Arctic Greenland. *American Journal of Tropical Medicine and Hygiene*, **10**, 185–190.

Opisthorchis felineus (Rivolta, 1884) Blanchard, 1895

DH: MAN; domesticated cat, dog and pig

IH1: *Bythnia* (*Bulimus*) *leachii* and *B. tentaculta* (snails)

IH2: Species of cyprinid fish including, *Abramis brama* (bream), *Barbus barbus* (barbel) and *Tinca tinca* (tench)

GD: Europe (USSR, Siberia); helminth distributed widely in central, eastern and southern Europe

LM: Liver, biliary system and lung

ND: Opisthorchiasis due to *Opisthorchis felineus*

TM: Ingestion of metacercaria with raw, salted or undercooked fish

Golyanitsakaya, O. N., 1945, Occurrence of *Opisthorchis felineus* in the human lung. *Problemi Tuberkuleza Moscow*, **3**, 57–58.

Opisthorchis guayaquilensis Rodriguez, Gomez, Lince and Montalvan, 1949

DH: MAN; domesticated cat and dog, *Canis latrans* (coyote)

IH1: Presumably species of snail

IH2: Presumably species of fish

GD: The Americas (Equador)

LM: Presumably biliary system. (Eggs have been recovered from a human stool)

ND: Opisthorchiasis due to *Opisthorchis guayaquilensis*

TM: Presumably ingestion of metacercaria

Artigas, P. de T. and Perez, M. D., 1960–1962, Consideracoes sobre *Opisthorchis pricei* Foster, 1939, *O. guayaquilensis* Rodriguez, Gomez et Montalvan 1949, e *O. pseudofelineus* Ward, 1901, Descricao de *Amphimerus pseudofelineus minitus* n.subsp. *Memorias do Instituto Butantan* (*Sao Paula*), **30**, 157–166.

Opisthorchis noverca Braun, 1903

DH: Man; domesticated dog and pig

IH1: Unresolved

IH2: Unresolved

GD: Asia (India)

LM: Gall bladder

ND: Opisthorchiasis due to *Opisthorchis noverca*

TM: Presumably ingestion of metacercaria

Leiper, R. T., 1913, Observations on certain helminths of man. *Transactions of the Royal Society of Tropical Medicine and Hygiene*, **6**, 265-297.

Opisthorchis sinensis (Cobbold, 1875) Blanchard, 1895

S: *Clonorchis sinensis*

DH: MAN; domesticated cat, dog and pig, species of piscivorous carnivore including *Martes* sp. (marten), *Meles meles* (badger) and *Mustela* spp. (mink and weasel)

IH1: *Bulimus striatulus japonicus*, *B. fushsianus* and *Parafossarulus manchouricus* (snails)

IH2: Numerous species of cyprinid fish

GD: Asia (China, Japan, Korea, Taiwan, North Vietnam)

LM: Liver, biliary system and pancreatic duct

ND: Clonorchiasis due to *Clonorchis sinensis*

TM: Ingestion of metacercaria with raw or undercooked fish

Komiya, Y., 1966, *Clonorchis* and Clonorchiasis. *Advances in Parasitology*, **4**, 53-106.

Opisthorchis viverrini (Poirier, 1886) Stiles and Hassall, 1896

DH: MAN; domesticated cat and dog; *Felis viverrinus* (civet cat) and various species of piscivorous mammal

IH1: *Bythnia funiculata, B. goniomphalus* and *B. laevis* (snails)

IH2: *Cyclocheilichthys siaja, Hampala dispar* and *Puntius orphoides* (freshwater fish)

GD: Asia (Laos, Thailand)

LM: Biliary system

ND: Opisthorchiasis due to *Opisthorchis viverrini*

TM: Ingestion of metacercaria with raw or undercooked fish

Harinasuta, C. and Harinasuta, T., 1984, *Opisthorchis viverrini*: life cycle, intermediate hosts, transmission to man and geographical distribution in Thailand. *Arzneimittel Forschung*, **34**, 1164–1167.

Pseudamphistomum aethiopicum Pierantoni, 1942

DH: Man

IH1: Unresolved

IH2: Unresolved

GD: Africa (Ethiopia)

LM: "Cyst-like" nodules from the internal wall of the small intestine

TM: Presumably ingestion of metacercaria

Cacciapuoti, R., 1947, Su di una nuova distomatosi umana en Ethiopia. *Riv. Biol. Cor. Roma.*, **8**, 111–116.

Pseudamphistomum truncatum (Rudolphi, 1819) Luhe, 1909

DH: MAN; domesticated cat and dog, *Mustela vison* (mink), *Phoca* sp. (seal) and *Vulpes vulpes* (fox)

IH1: Unresolved

IH2: Species of freshwater fish including *Abramis brama* (bream) and *Carassius auratus* (goldfish)

GD: Europe (USSR)

LM: Liver

TM: Ingestion of metacercaria with raw, salted or undercooked fish

Vinogradov, K. N., 1982, On a new species of distome (*Distomum sibircum*) in the human liver. *Izvest. Imp. Tomsk University*, **4**, 116-160.

HETEROPHYIDAE

Apophallus donicus (Skrjabin and Lindtrop, 1919) Price, 1931

DH: MAN; domesticated cat and dog, rabbit, *Vulpes vulpes* (red fox) and species of bird including *Nycticorax* sp. (heron)

IH1: *Flumenicola virens* (snail)

IH2: Species of fish including *Richardsonius balteatus* (redside shiner), *Ptychocheilus oregonensis* (squaw fish) and *Salmo gairdneri* (rainbow trout)

GD: The Americas (Canada)

LM: Small intestine; "Eggs typical of this species were found in the feces of . . ."

TM: Ingestion of metacercaria (experimental)

Niemi, D. R. and Macy, R. W., 1974, The life cycle and infectivity to man of *Apophallus donicus* (Skrjabin and Lindtrop, 1919) (Trematoda: Heterophyidae) in Oregon. *Proceedings of the Helminthological Society of Washington*, **41**, 223-229.

Centrocestus armatus (Tanabe, 1922)

DH: Man (experimental); domesticated cat and dog, species of piscivorous bird including *Nycticorax nycticorax* (night heron), *Ardea cinerea* (grey heron) and *Egretta i. intermedia* (egret)

IH1: *Semisulcospira libertina* and *S. multigranosa* (snails)

IH2: Several species of cyprinid fish

GD: Asia (Japan)

LM: Presumably small intestine

TM: Ingestion of metacercaria with raw or undercooked second intermediate host

Ulmer, M. J., 1975, Other trematode infections. In *Diseases Transmitted from Animals to Man*, edited by W. T. Hubbert, W. F. McCulloch and P. R. Schnurrenberger, (Springfield, Illinois: C. C. Thomas) pp. 646–677.

Centrocestus formosanus Nishigori, 1924

DH: Man; domesticated cat and dog, rat and several species of piscivorous bird including *Egretta i. intermedia* (egret)

IH1: Species of *Semisulcospira* and *Melania* (snails)

IH2: Several species of brackish and freshwater fish, also species of *Rana* (frog) and *Bufo* (toad)

GD: Asia (Japan)

LM: Small intestine

TM: Ingestion of metacercaria with raw or undercooked second intermediate host

Komiya, Y. and Suzuki, N., 1966, Metacercariae of trematodes of the family Heterophyidae from Japan and adjacent countries. *Japanese Journal of Parasitology*, **15**, 208–214.

Cryptocotyle lingua (Creplin, 1825)

DH: MAN; domesticated cat and dog, species of piscivorous mammal and bird

IH1: Species of *Tautogolabrus* (snails)

IH2: Species of fish including *Gobius ruthensparri* (two-spotted goby) and *Pleuronectes platessa* (plaice)

GD: The Americas (Greenland)

LM: Presumably small intestine; "Eggs ... were found in ... faecal samples ..."

TM: Ingestion of metacercaria with raw or undercooked fish

Rausch, R. L., Scott, E. M. and Rausch, V. R., 1967, Helminths in Eskimos in Western Alaska, with particular reference to *Diphyllobothrium* infection and anaemia. *Transactions of the Royal Society of Tropical Medicine and Hygiene*, **61**, 351–357.

Haplorchis pumilio (Looss, 1896) Looss, 1899

DH: MAN; domesticated cat and dog, species of piscivorous bird including *Larus milvus* (seagull), *Nycticorax nycticorax* (night heron) and *Pelecanus onocrotalus* (pelican)

IH1: *Melania reiniana* and *M. tuberculata* (snails)

IH2: Several species of fish including *Puntius binotatus* (barbin)

GD: Africa (Egypt); Asia (Philippines)

LM: Presumably small intestine; "... eggs tentatively diagnosed ... in sections of the spinal cord ..." (Beaver *et al.*, 1984, *Clinical Parasitology*, p. 481)

TM: Ingestion of metacercaria with raw or undercooked fish

Africa, C. M. and Garcia, E. Y., 1935, Heterophyid trematodes of man and dogs in the Philippines with descriptions of three new species. *Philippine Journal of Science*, **57**, 253–268.

Haplorchis taichui (Nishigori, 1924)

DH: MAN; domesticated cat and dog, cattle

IH1: *Melania obliquegranosa* and *Melanoides tubercultus* (snails)

IH2: Species of fish including *Puntius leiacanthus, P. gonionotus* and *P. orphoides* (barbins)

GD: Africa (Egypt); Asia (Philippines)

LM: Presumably small intestine; cardiac involvement, "... valvular enlargement ... with presence of eggs ..." (Ulmer, 1975, In *Diseases Transmitted from Animals to Man*, p. 656)

TM: Ingestion of metacercaria with raw or undercooked fish

Tadros, G. and El-Mokaddem, E. E. A., 1983, Observations on heterophyids affecting man in Egypt. *Bulletin of the Zoological Society of Egypt*, **33**, 107–111.

Haplorchis vanissimus Africa, 1938

DH: MAN; species of piscivorous bird including *Haliastur sphenurus* (whistling eagle), *Nycticorax caledonius* (heron) and *Phalacrocorax ater* (cormorant)

IH1: Presumably species of snail

IH2: Presumably species of fish

GD: Asia (Philippines, Bohol Island)

LM: Small intestine

TM: Presumably ingestion of metacercaria

Africa, C. M., 1938, Description of three trematodes of the genus *Haplorchis* (Heterophyidae) with notes on two other members of the genus. *Philippine Journal of Science*, **66**, 299–307.

Haplorchis yokogawai (Katsuta, 1932)

DH: MAN; domesticated cat and dog, cattle, *Macacus cynomolgus* (crab-eating macaque) and species of piscivorous bird including *Ardea purpurea manilensis* (purple heron), *Haliastur indus* (Brahminy kite) and *Strix whiteheadi* (owl)

IH1:   *Stenomelania newcombi* (snail)

IH2:   Species of fish including *Cirrhina reba*, *Ophicephalus striatus* and *Puntius sarana*

GD: Africa (Egypt); The Americas (USA, Hawaii); Asia (Indonesia, Philippines)

LM: Small intestine

TM: Ingestion of metacercaria with raw or undercooked fish

Kwo Eh Hoa and Lie-Kian Joe., 1953, Occurrence in man in Indonesia of trematodes commonly found in animals. *Journal Indonesian Medical Association*, **3**, 131–136.

Heterophyes dispar Looss, 1902

DH: MAN; domesticated cat and dog, *Vulpes vulpes* (red fox) and species of piscivorous mammal

IH1:   *Pirenella conica* (snail)

IH2:   Species of fish including *Barbus canis*, *Mugil cephalus* (mullet), *Sciaena aquilla* (Atlantic shade fish) and *Solea vulgaris* (sole)

GD: Asia (Korea)

LM: Small intestine; "The stool examination revealed heterophyid eggs ..."

ND: Heterophyiasis due to *Heterophyes dispar*

TM: Ingestion of metacercaria with raw or undercooked fish

Chai, J. Y., Seo, B. S., Lee, S. H., Hong, S. J. and Sohn, W. M., 1986, Human infections by *Heterophyes heterophyes* and *H. dispar* imported from Saudi Arabia. *Korean Journal of Parasitology*, **24**, 82–88.

Heterophyes heterophyes (v. Siebold, 1852) Stiles and Hassall, 1900

DH: MAN; domesticated cat and dog, *Vulpes vulpes* (fox) and species of piscivorous mammal

IH1: *Pirenella conica* (Egypt) and *Cerithidea cingulata* (Japan) (snails)

IH2: Species of fish including *Aphanius fasciatus*, *Mugil cephalus* (mullet) and *Tilapia nilotica* (nile perch)

GD: Africa (Egypt); Asia (Japan, Korea); Europe (France)

LM: Small intestine; also, "Egg and/or worm granuloma, presumably due to ... from the human brain ... a pulmonary complication..."

ND: Heterophyiasis due to *Heterophyes heterophyes*

TM: Ingestion of metacercaria with raw, salted or undercooked fish

Chai, J. Y., Seo, B. S., Lee, S. H., Hong, S. J. and Sohn, W. M., 1986, Human infections by *Heterophyes heterophyes* and *H. dispar* imported from Saudi Arabia. *Korean Journal of Parasitology*, **24**, 82–88.

Heterophyes nocens Onji and Nishio, 1916

DH: MAN

IH1: Presumably species of snail

IH2: Species of fish including *Acanthogobius flavimanus* (goby), *Lateolabrax japonicus* (perch) and *Mugil cephalus* (mullet)

GD: Asia (Japan, Korea)

LM: Small intestine; "... heart arrhythmia, suggesting an erratic parasitism in the heart."

ND: Heterophyiasis due to *Heterophyes heterophyes nocens*

TM: Ingestion of metacercaria with raw, salted or undercooked fish

Chai, J. Y., Hong, S. J., Sohn, W. M., Lee, S. H. and Seo, B. S., 1985. Further cases of human *Heterophyes heterophyes nocens* infection in Korea. *Seoul Journal of Medicine*, **26**, 197–200.

Heterophyopsis continua (Onji and Nishio, 1916) Price, 1940

DH: MAN; domesticated cat and dog

IH1:   Possibly *Cerithidea angulata* (snail)

IH2:   Species of fish including *Acanthogobius flavimanus* (goby), *Lateolabrax japonicus* (perch) and *Mugil cephalus* (mullet)

GD: Asia (Japan, Korea)

LM: Small intestine; "... examination of the successive diarrheal stools 46 specimens of *H. continua* ..." ... "... possibility that ... may cause cardiac heterophyidiasis ..."

TM: Ingestion of metacercaria with raw, salted or undercooked fish

Seo, B. S., Lee, S. H., Chai, J. Y. and Hong, S. J., 1984, Studies on intestinal trematodes in Korea XIII. Two cases of natural human infection by *Heterophyopsis continua* and the status of metacercarial infection in brackish water fishes. *Korean Journal of Parasitology*, **22**, 51–60.

Metagonimus minutis Katsuta, 1932

DH: MAN; domesticated cat, mouse (experimental)

IH1:   Presumably species of snail

IH2:   Fish

GD: Asia (Taiwan)

LM: Small intestine

TM: Ingestion of metacercaria with raw or undercooked fish

Bunnag, D. and Harinasuta, T., 1986, Intestinal trematodiases. Unpublished communication to W.H.O. Expert Committee Meeting, Geneva, March 1986.

Metagonimus yokogawai (Katsurada, 1912) Katsurada, 1913

DH: MAN; domesticated cat and dog, rat, many species of piscivorous bird

IH1: *Semisulcospira libertina* and *S. coreana* (snails)

IH2: Species of cyprinid fish including *Plecoglossus altivelis* (sweet fish)

GD: Asia (China, Indonesia, Japan, Korea, Philippines, Taiwan)

LM: Small intestine, intimately associated with the mucosa

ND: Metagonimiasis due to *Metagonimus yokogawai*

TM: Ingestion of metacercaria with raw, salted or undercooked fish

Cho, S. Y., Kang, S. Y. and Lee, J. B., 1984, Metagonimiasis in Korea. *Arzneimittel-Forschung Drug Research*, **34**, 1211–1213.

Procerovum calderoni (Africa and Garcia, 1935) Price, 1940

DH: MAN; (experimental in cat, dog and chicken)

IH1: *Melania tuberculata chinensis* and *Thiara riquetti* (snails)

IH2: Species of fish including *Butis amboinensis*, *Chanos chanos*, *Mugil dussumieri*, *Ophicephalus striatus* and *Platycephalus indicus*

GD: Asia (Philippines)

LM: Small intestine

TM: Ingestion of metacercaria with raw, salted or undercooked fish

Africa, C. M., 1938, Description of three trematodes of the genus *Haplorchis* (Heterophyidae) with notes on two other Philippine members of this genus. *Philippine Journal of Science*, **66**, 299–307.

Procerovum varium Onji and Nishio, 1916

DH: MAN (experimental); domesticated dog and *Nycticorax caledonicus* (rufus night heron)

IH1: Presumably species of snail

IH2: Species of fish including *Glossamia aprion*

GD: Asia (Japan)

LM: Presumably alimentary tract; "... eggs were recovered ... after human subjects swallowed metacercariae ..." (Ulmer, 1975, In *Diseases Transmitted from Animals to Man*, p. 659.)

TM: Experimental ingestion of metacercaria

Aokage, K., 1956, Studies on the trematode parasites of brackish water fishes in Chugoku coast of Setonaikai. *Tokyo Iji Shinshi*, **73**, 217-224.

Pygidiopsis summa Onji and Nishio, 1916

DH: MAN; domesticated cat and dog, experimentally in mouse, rabbit and rat, species of piscivorous bird including *Milvus migrans lineatus* (black-eared kite) and *Nyctocorax nyctocorax* (night heron)

IH1: *Tympanotonus microptera* (snail)

IH2: Species of fish including *Acanthogobius flavimanus* (goby), *Liza menada* and *Mugil cephalus* (mullet)

GD: Asia (Korea)

LM: Small intestine; "... eggs ... during stool examination ... all the cases ... adult worms after treatment ..."

TM: Ingestion of metacercaria with raw, salted or undercooked fish

Seo, B. S., Hong, S. T. and Chai, J. Y., 1981, Studies on intestinal trematodes in Korea III. Natural human infections of *Pygidiopsis summa* and *Heterophyes heterophyes nocens*. *Social Journal of Medicine*, **22**, 228-235.

Stellantchasmus falcatus Onji and Nishio, 1916

DH: MAN; domesticated cat and dog, rat and species of piscivorous bird including *Colymbus arcticus pacificus* (diver)

IH1: *Stenomelania newcombi* and *Thiara granifera* (snails)

IH2: Species of fish including *Acanthogobius flavimanus* (goby), *Liza menada* and *Mugil cephalus* (mullet)

GD: The Americas (USA, Hawaii); Asia (Japan, Korea, Philippines, Thailand)

LM: Presumably alimentary tract; "... from diarrheal stools ... flukes [adult] were collected ..."

TM: Ingestion of metacercaria with raw, salted or undercooked fish

Seo, B. S., Lee, S. H., Chai, Y. L. and Hong, S. J., 1984, Studies on intestinal trematodes in Korea XII. Two cases of human infection by *Stellantchasmus falcatus*. *Korean Journal of Parasitology*, **22**, 43–50.

Stictodora fuscata Onji and Nishio, 1916

DH: MAN; species of piscivorous bird

IH1: Presumably species of snail.

IH2: Presumably species of brackish water fish.

GD: Asia (Korea).

LM: Presumably alimentary tract; "Two adult specimens ... genus *Stictodora* ... collected from the stool ... after chemotherapy."

TM: Presumably ingestion of metacercaria with raw, salted or undercooked fish.

Chai, Y. L., Hong, S. J., Lee, S. H. and Seo, B. S., 1988, *Stictodora* sp. (Trematoda: Heterophyidae) recovered from a man in Korea. *Korean Journal of Parasitology*, **26**, 127–132.

MICROPHALLIDAE

Carneophallus brevicaeca (Africa and Garcia, 1935) Velasquez 1975

S: *Spelotrema brevicaeca, Heterophyes brevicaeca*

DH: MAN; *Macacus irus* (macaque monkey) and *Sterna albifrons sinensis* (tern)

IH1: Unresolved

IH2: *Macrobrachium* sp. (shrimp)

GD: Asia (Philippines)

LM: Presumably alimentary tract; "... eggs have been found in cardiac muscles of patients at autopsy." (Ulmer, 1975, In *Diseases Transmitted from Animals to Man*, p. 656)

TM: Ingestion of metacercaria

Africa, C. M. and Garcia, E. Y., 1935, Heterophyid trematodes of man and dogs in the Philippines with descriptions of three new species. *Philippine Journal of Science*, **57**, 253–268.

Microphallus minus Ochi, 1928

DH: MAN (experimental); domesticated dog, rat, experimentally in cat, mouse and rat

IH1: Unresolved

IH2: *Macrobrachium* sp. (shrimp)

GD: Asia (Japan)

LM: Presumably small intestine

TM: Ingestion of metacercaria

Ochi, S., 1928, On a new trematode *Microphallus* n. sp. which has long-legged shrimp as intermediate host. *Tokyo Iji Shinshi* (2587): 1363–1370. Abstract in *Japanese Journal of Zoology*.

Isoparorchis hypselobagri (Billet, 1898) Odhner, 1927

DH: Man; adult worms commonly in swim bladder of species of freshwater (siluroid) fish

IH1: *Posticobia brazieri* (experimental) (snail)

IH2: Unresolved; probably a small crustacean*

GD: Asia (China, India); helminth widely distributed in Asia and Oceania in fish hosts

LM: Presumably alimentary tract; "... fluke recovered from the stool of a human patient ... given an anthelmintic ..." (Ulmer, 1975, In *Diseases Transmitted from Animals to Man*, p. 660)

TM: Ingestion of metacercaria with raw or undercooked fish

Chandler, A. C., 1926, The prevalence and epidemiology of hookworm and other helmintic infections in India IV. *Indian Journal of Medical Research*, **14**, 481–492.

CESTOIDEA

EUCESTODA

TRYPANORHYNCA

TENTACULARIIDAE

Nybelinia surmenicola Okada, 1929

DH: Man

IH: Species of cephalopod mollusc including *Ommastrephes solani pacificus* (squid)

GD: Asia (Japan)

*Cribb, T. H., 1988, Two new digenetic trematodes from Australian fishes with notes on previously described species. *Journal of Natural History*, **22**, 27–43.

LM: "... larva was found tightly attaching itself ... to his left palative tonsil ..."

TM: Presumably ingestion of larva with raw squid

Kikuchi, V., Takenouchi, T., Kamiya, M. and Ozaki, H., 1981, Trypanorhynchiid cestode larva found on the human palative tonsil. *Japanese Journal of Parasitology*, **30**, 497–499.

PSEUDOPHYLLIDEA

DIPHYLLOBOTHRIIDAE

Diphyllobothrium cameroni Rausch, 1969

DH: MAN; *Monachus schauinslandi* (Hawaiian monk seal)

IH1: Presumably species of copepod

IH2: Presumably species of marine fish

GD: Asia (Japan)

LM: Small intestine; "... spontaneously expelled ... mature proglottids ..."

ND: Diphyllobothriasis due to *Diphyllobothrium cameroni*

TM: Presumably ingestion of plerocercoid with raw, salted or undercooked fish

Kamo, H., Yamane, Y. and Kawashima, K., 1981, The first record of human infection with *Diphyllobothrium cameroni* Rausch, 1969. *Japanese Journal of Tropical Medicine and Hygiene*, **9**, 199–205.

Diphyllobothrium cordatum Cobbold, 1879

DH: MAN; domesticated dog and *Erignathus barbatus* (common bearded seal), *Odabaenus rosmarus* (walrus) and *Phoca groenlandica* (harp seal)

IH1: Presumably species of copepod

IH2: Presumably species of marine fish

GD: The Americas (USA, Alaska)

LM: Small intestine

ND: Diphyllobothriasis due to *Diphyllobothrium cordatum*

TM: Presumably ingestion of plerocercoid with raw, salted or undercooked fish

Rausch, R. L., Scott, E. M. and Rausch, V. R., 1967, Helminths in Eskimos in Western Alaska with a particular reference to *Diphyllobothrium* infection and anaemia. *Transactions of the Royal Society of Tropical Medicine and Hygiene*, **61**, 351–357.

Diphyllobothrium dalliae Rausch, 1956

DH: MAN; domesticated dog, *Alopex lagopus* (arctic fox) and species of seagull

IH1: Presumably species of copepod

IH2: Species of freshwater fish including *Dallia pectoralis* (blackfish)

GD: The Americas (USA, Alaska)

LM: Small intestine; "... a common parasite of man ... From one resident ... in addition to 16 well-developed adult cestodes, ..."

ND: Diphyllobothriasis due to *Diphyllobothrium dalliae*

TM: Ingestion of plerocercoid with raw, salted or undercooked fish

Rausch, R. L. and Hilliard, D. K., 1970, Studies on the helminth fauna of Alaska XLIX. The occurrence of *Diphyllobothrium latum* (Linnaeus, 1758) (Cestoda: Diphyllobothriidae) in Alaska, with notes on other species. *Canadian Journal of Zoology*, **48**, 1201–1219.

Diphyllobothrium dendriticum (Nitzsch, 1824)

DH: MAN; domesticated cat and dog, species of piscivorous bird including *Larus ridibundus* (black-headed gull)

IH1: Species of copepod including *Cyclops strenuus*, *Diaptomus gracilis* and *D. graciloides*

IH2: Species of freshwater fish including *Lota lota* (burbot) and *Salmo gairdneri* (rainbow trout)

GD: The Americas (USA, Alaska)

LM: Small intestine; "Strobilae ... have been obtained ... and from man in Alaska."

ND: Diphyllobothriasis due to *Diphyllobothrium dendriticum*

TM: Ingestion of plerocercoid with raw, salted or undercooked fish

Rausch, R. L. and Hilliard, D. K., 1970, Studies on the helminth fauna of Alaska XLIX. The occurrence of *Diphyllobothrium latum* (Linnaeus, 1758) (Cestoda: Diphyllobothriidae) in Alaska, with notes on other species. *Canadian Journal of Zoology*, **48**, 1201–1219.

Diphyllobothrium elegans (Krabbe, 1865)

DH: Man; *Phoca crista* and *P. vitulina* (seals), *Eumetopias jubata* (steller sea lion)

IH1: Presumably species of copepod

IH2: Presumably species of marine fish

GD: Asia (Japan)

LM: Small intestine ... "specimens from man ... some of which are similar to *Diphyllobothrium elegans*".

ND: Diphyllobothriasis due to *Diphyllobothrium elegans*

TM: Presumably ingestion of plerocercoid with raw, salted or undercooked fish

Kamo, H., 1978, The occurrence of human infections with some marine species of *Diphyllobothrium* in Japan. Short communication, *4th International Congress of Parasitology*, Section B, 30 Abstract.

Diphyllobothrium erinaceieuropaei (Rudolphi, 1819)

DH: MAN; species of carnivorous mammal including domesticated cat and dog

IH1: Presumably species of copepod

IH2: Presumably species of fish

GD: Asia (Japan); helminth widely distributed in species of carnivorous mammal

LM: Small intestine; "A strobila without scolex was spontaneously discharged ... egg ..."

ND: Diphyllobothriasis due to *Diphyllobothrium erinaceieuropaei*

TM: Presumably ingestion of plerocercoid with raw, salted or undercooked fish

Suzuki, N., Kumazawa, H., Hosogi, H. and Nakagawa, O., 1982, A case of human infection with the adult of *Spirometra erinacei* (Rudolphi, 1819) Faust, Campbell and Kellogg, 1929. *Japanese Journal of Parasitology*, **31**, 23–26.

Diphyllobothrium giljacicum Rutkevich, 1937

DH: Man

IH1: Presumably species of copepod

IH2: Presumably species of fish

GD: Europe (USSR)

LM: Presumably small intestine

ND: Diphyllobothriasis due to *Diphyllobothrium giljacicum*

TM: Presumably ingestion of plerocercoid with raw or undercooked fish

Rutkevich, N. L., 1937, *Diphyllobothrium giljacicum* nov. sp. and *Diphyllobothrium luxi* n. sp. two new tapeworms of man from Sakhalin. *Rab. Gel'mintol* Skrjabin, 574–580.

Diphyllobothrium hians (Diesing, 1850)

DH: MAN; *Monachus monachus* (Mediterranean monk seal), *Phoca mona-drus, P. hispida* and *P. barbata* (seals)

IH1: Presumably species of copepod

IH2: Presumably species of marine fish

GD: Europe (USSR, Amur River)

LM: "On physical examination ulceration was noted on the lesser curvature of the stomach ... orally administered bithionol ... expelled a worm about 70 cm long. ... gravid uterus. Eggs ..."

ND: Diphyllobothriasis due to *Diphyllobothrium hians*

TM: Presumably ingestion of plerocercoid with raw, salted or undercooked marine fish

Kamo, H., Yazaki, S., Fukumoto, S., Fujino, T., Koga, M., Ishii, Y. and Matsuo, E., 1988, The first human case infected with *Diphyllobothrium hians* (Diesing, 1850). *Japanese Journal of Parasitology*, **37**, 29–35.

Diphyllobothrium klebanovskii Muratov and Posokhov, 1988

DH: MAN; hamster (experimental)

IH1: Presumably species of copepod

IH2: Species of salmon including *Oncorhynchus keta* and *O. gorbusha*

GD: Europe (USSR, Amur River)

LM: Small intestine; "... of 51 specimens expelled from men ..."

ND: Diphyllobothriasis due to *Diphyllobothrium klebanovskii*

TM: Ingestion of plerocercoid with raw, salted or undercooked fish

Muratov, I. V. and Posokhov, P. S., 1988, *Diphyllobothrium klebanovskii* sp. n. a parasite of man. *Parazitologiya Akademiya Nauk* SSR Leningrad, **22**, 165–170.

Diphyllobothrium lanceolatum (Krabbe, 1865)

DH: Man; domesticated dog, *Phoca barbata* and *P. vitulina* (seals)

IH1:   Presumably species of copepod

IH2:   Presumably species of fish including *Coregonus sardinella* (whitefish)

GD: The Americas (USA, Alaska)

LM: Small intestine; "From a resident of Chevak, treated with quinacrine ... were obtained among which was a single plerocercoid of *D. lanceolatum.*"

TM: Presumably ingestion of plerocercoid in raw, salted or undercooked fish

Rausch, R. L. and Hilliard, D. K., 1970, Studies on the helminth fauna of Alaska XLIX. The occurrence of *Diphyllobothrium latum* (Linnaeus, 1758) (Cestoda: Diphyllobothriidae) in Alaska, with notes on other species. *Canadian Journal of Zoology*, **48**, 1201-1209.

Diphyllobothrium latum (Linnaeus, 1758) Cobbold, 1858

DH: MAN; domesticated dog, species of *Ursus* (bears) and many species of piscivorous mammals

IH1:   Species of fresh water copepod including *Diaptomus vulgaris*, *D. gracilis* and *Cyclops vicinus*

IH2:   Numerous species of freshwater fish including *Esox lucius* (pike), *Perca fluviatilis* (perch) and *Lota lota* (burbot)

GD: Widely distributed in subarctic temperate regions

LM: Small intestine

ND: Diphyllobothriasis due to *Diphyllobothrium latum*

TM: Ingestion of plerocercoid with raw, salted or undercooked fish

von Bonsdorff, B., 1978, The broad tapeworm story. *Acta Medica Scandinavia*, **204**, 241-247.

Diphyllobothrium mansoni (Cobbold, 1882) Mueller, 1937

DH: Domesticated cat and dog

IH1: Species of *Cyclops* (Copepoda)

IH2: MAN; various species of freshwater fish, *Rana nigromaculata* (frog); species of snake including *Dinodon rufozonatum*, *Elaphe schrenckii* and *Natrix tigrina*; experimentally in guinea-pig, mouse, rabbit and rat

GD: Asia (China, Hong Kong, Japan, North Korea, South Korea)

LM: Plerocercoid (sparganum) in subcutaneous tissue, muscle tissue and CNS

ND: Spirometrosis (sparganosis) due to *Diphyllobothrium mansoni*

TM: Ingestion of procercoid in copepod in contaminated drinking water. Ingestion of plerocercoid with raw or undercooked second intermediate host. Application of a poultice to a wound or abscess using infected flesh of second intermediate host.

Ng, T. H. K., Wong, W. T., Fund, C. F. and Leung, C. Y., 1989, Clinical sparganosis in Hong Kong. *Journal of the Royal Society of Health*, **4**, 138–140.

Diphyllobothrium mansonoides Mueller, 1935

S: *Spirometra mansonoides*

DH: Domesticated cat and dog, *Procyon lotor* (raccoon) and various species of carnivorous mammal

IH1: Species of *Cyclops* including *C. vernalis*

IH2: MAN; species of frog (adult and tadpole) and species of snake including *Natrix natrix* (water snake)

GD: The Americas (Canada, USA)

LM: Plerocercoid (sparganum) found in subcutaneous and other tissues

ND: Spirometrosis (sparganosis) due to *Diphyllobothrium mansonoides*

TM: Ingestion of procercoid in *Cyclops* species contaminating drinking water

Mueller, J. F., 1974, The biology of *Spirometra*. *Journal of Parasitology*, **60**, 3–14.

Diphyllobothrium minus Cholodkovsky, 1916

DH: MAN; domesticated cat and dog, seagulls

IH1: Presumably species of copepod

IH2: Presumably species of fish

GD: Europe (USSR)

LM: Small intestine; specimen (stobila and eggs) passed after anthelmintic treatment

TM: Presumably ingestion of plerocercoid with raw, salted or undercooked fish

Cholodkovsky, N., 1916, Abstracted in *Tropical Diseases Bulletin*, 19, 669 (1922).

Diphyllobothrium nenzi Petrov, 1938

DH: MAN

IH1: Presumably species of copepod

IH2: Presumably species of fish

GD: Europe (USSR)

LM: Small intestine

TM: Presumably ingestion of plerocercoid with raw, salted or undercooked fish

Petrov, M. I., 1938, New diphyllobothriids of man. *Medical Parasitology and Parasitic Disease*, **7**, 406–413.

Diphyllobothrium nihonkaiense Yamane, Kamo, Bylund and Wikgren, 1986

DH: MAN

IH1: Presumably species of copepod

IH2: Species of salmon including *Oncorhynchus gorbuscha* and *O. masou*

GD: Asia (Japan)

LM: Small intestine

ND: Diphyllobothriasis due to *Diphyllobothrium nihonkaiense*

TM: Ingestion of plerocercoid with raw, salted or undercooked fish

Fukumoto, S., Yazaki, S., Kamo, H., Yamane, Y. and Tsuji, M., 1988, Distinction between *Diphyllobothrium nihonkaiense* and *Diphyllobothrium latum* by immunoelectrophoresis. *Japanese Journal of Parasitology*, **37**, 91–95.

Diphyllobothrium pacificum (Nybelin, 1931) Margolis, 1956

DH: MAN; species of marine mammal including *Callorhinus ursinus* (fur seal) and *Otaria flavescens* (sea lion)

IH1: Presumably species of copepod

IH2: Species of marine fish including *Sarda chilensis* and *Scomberomorus maculatus* (mackerel)

GD: The Americas (Peru); Asia (Japan)

LM: Small intestine; "Strobila of a tapeworm ... expelled from a 54-year-old seaman ... eggs hatched in sea water ..."

ND: Diphyllobothriasis due to *Diphyllobothrium pacificum*

TM: Ingestion of plerocercoid with raw, salted or undercooked fish

Makiya, K., Tsukamoto, M., Horio, M. and Goto, M., 1987, *Diphyllobothrium pacificum*, a cestode of marine mammals, expelled from a Japanese seaman. *Japanese Journal of Parasitology*, **36**, 145–153.

Diphyllobothrium scoticum (Rennie and Reid, 1912)

DH: MAN; *Hydrurga leptonyx* (leopard seal) and *Otaria byronica* (South American sea lion)

IH1:   Presumably species of copepod

IH2:   Presumably species of fish

GD: Asia (Japan)

LM: Small intestine: "A strobila was expelled from a seaman ... after the treatment with bithionol ... mature and gravid segments ..."

ND: Diphyllobothriasis due to *Diphyllobothrium scoticum*

TM: Presumably ingestion of plerocercoid with raw, salted or undercooked fish

Fukumoto, S., Yazaki, S., Maejima, J., Kamo, H., Takao, Y. and Tsutsumi, H., 1988, The first report of human infection with *Diphyllobothrium scoticum* (Rennie and Reid, 1912). *Japanese Journal of Parasitology*, **37**, 84–90.

Diphyllobothrium skrjabini Plotnikov, 1932

DH: MAN; domesticated dog

IH1:   Presumably species of copepod

IH2:   Presumably species of fish

GD: Europe (USSR)

LM: Small intestine

ND: Diphyllobothriasis due to *Diphyllobothrium skrjabini*

TM: Presumably ingestion of plerocercoid with raw, salted or undercooked fish

Petrov, M. I., 1938, New diphyllobothriids of man. *Medical Parasitology and Parasitic Disease*, **7**, 406–413.

Diphyllobothrium theileri Baer, 1925

DH: Species of carnivorous mammal in Africa including *Crocuta crocuta* (spotted hyena)

IH1: Species of copepod

IH2: MAN; species of wild herbivorous mammal

GD: Africa (Kenya)

LM: Plerocercoid found in subcutaneous tissue

ND: Spirometrosis (sparganosis) due to *Diphyllobothrium theileri*

TM: Ingestion of procercoid in copepod contaminating drinking water

Baer, J. G., 1974, Problems d'epidemiologie de quelques cestodes de l'homme. *Parassitologia*, **16**, 47–52.

Diphyllobothrium tungussicum Podjapolskaia and Gnedina, 1932

DH: MAN

IH1: Presumably species of copepod

IH2: Presumably species of fish

GD: Europe (USSR)

LM: Small intestine

ND: Diphyllobothriasis due to *Diphyllobothrium tungussicum*

TM: Presumably ingestion of plerocercoid with raw, salted or undercooked fish

Podjapolskaia, V. P. and Gnedina, M. P., 1932, *Diphyllobothrium tungussicum* n. sp. ein neuer Parasit des Menschen. *Centrablatt fur Bakteriologie und Parasitenkunde,* **126**, 415-419.

Diphyllobothrium ursi Rausch, 1954

DH: MAN; *Ursus americanus* (black bear) and *U. arctos* (brown bear)

IH1:   Species of copepod

IH2:   Species of fish including *Oncorhynchus nerka* (red salmon)

GD: The Americas (Canada; USA, Alaska)

LM: Small intestine

ND: Diphyllobothriasis due to *Diphyllobothrium ursi*

TM: Ingestion of plerocercoid with raw, salted or undercooked fish

Margolis, L., Rausch, R. L. and Robertson, E., 1973, *Diphyllobothrium ursi* from man in British Columbia—first report of this tapeworm in Canada. *Canadian Journal of Public Health,* **64**, 588-589.

Diphyllobothrium yonagoensis Yamane, Kamo, Yazaki, Fukumoto and Mae-jima, 1981

DH: MAN

IH1:   Presumably species of copepod

IH2:   Presumably species of fish

GD: Asia (Japan)

LM: Small intestine; "... expelled after treatment with Kamala ..."

ND: Diphyllobothriasis due to *Diphyllobothrium yonagoensis*

TM: Presumably ingestion of plerocercoid with raw, salted or undercooked fish

Kamo, H., Maejima, J., Yazaki, S., Fukumoto, S. and Yamanishi, Y., 1988, Human infection with *Diphyllobothrium yonagoensis* in Kinki-Tokai districts. *Japanese Journal of Parasitology*, **37**, 62–66.

Diplogonoporus balaenopterae Lönnberg, 1892

S: *Diplogonoporus grandis*

DH: MAN; domesticated dog, species of *Balaenoptera* including *B. borealis* (sei whale) and *B. acutorostrata* (lesser rorqual whale)

IH1:   Species of copepod including *Oithona nana* (experimental)

IH2:   Species of marine fish, probably *Engraulis japonicus* (anchovy) and *Sardinops melanostica* (sardine)

GD: Asia (Japan)

LM: Small intestine

TM: Presumably ingestion of plerocercoid with raw, salted or undercooked fish

Kamo, H., Hatsushika, R. and Yamane, Y., 1971, Diplogonoporiasis and diplogonadic cestodes in Japan. *Yonago Acta Medica*, **15**, 234–246.

Diplogonoporus brauni Leon, 1907

DH: Man; probably species of piscivorous bird

IH1:   Unresolved

IH2:   Presumably species of fish

GD: Europe (Romania)

LM: Small intestine

TM: Presumably ingestion of plerocercoid with raw, salted or undercooked fish

Joyeux, C. E. and Baer, J. G., 1929, Les cestodes rares de l'homme. *Bulletin Societe Pathologie Exotique*, **22**, 114-136.

Diplogonoporus fukuokaensis Kamo and Miyazaki, 1970

DH: MAN; presumably species of piscivorous mammal

IH1: Unresolved

IH2: Presumably species of fish

GD: Asia (Japan)

LM: Small intestine; "... was treated with 'kamala' ... evacuation on two occasions, containing a strobila with scolex ..."

TM: Presumably ingestion of plerocercoid with raw, salted or undercooked fish

Kamo, H. and Miyazaki, I., 1970, *Diplogonoporus fukuokaensis* sp. nov. (Cestoda; Diphyllobothriidae) from a girl in Japan. *Japanese Journal of Parasitology*, **19**, 635-644.

Ligula intestinalis (Linnaeus, 1758) Bloch, 1782

DH: Man; species of piscivorous bird

IH1: Species of copepod including *Cyclops strenuus, Diaptomus gracilis* and *Mesocyclops leuckarti*

IH2: Species of freshwater fish of the family Cyprinidae

GD: Europe (Poland, Romania)

LM: Presumably small intestine

TM: Presumably from ingestion of plerocercoid with raw or undercooked fish

Joyeux, C. E. and du Noyer, R., 1931, Presence d'une larve de ligule dans des vomissements. *Marseille Medical*, **68**, 235-236.

Pyramicocephalus anthocephalus (Fabricius, 1780) Monticelli, 1890

DH: MAN; domesticated dog, species of piscivorous mammal including *Phoca barbata* (bearded seal)

IH1: Unresolved

IH2: Species of marine fish including *Eliginus gracilis* (cod) and *Megalocottus platycephalus* (sculpin)

GD: The Americas (Greenland; USA, Alaska)

LM: Presumably small intestine

TM: Presumably ingestion of plerocercoid with raw, salted or undercooked fish

Schmidt, G. D., 1986, *CRC Handbook of Tapeworm Identification* (Boca Raton, Florida: CRC Press Inc.) 675 pp. (see pp. 91–92).

Schistocephalus solidus (Mueller, 1776) Creplin, 1829

DH: MAN; domesticated dog, species of piscivorous bird, experimentally in chicken, duck, hamster, pigeon and rat

IH1: Species of copepod including *Cyclops viridus* (experimental)

IH2: Species of freshwater fish including *Gasterosteus aculeatus* (three-spined stickleback)

GD: The Americas (USA, Alaska); helminth distributed worldwide

LM: Small intestine; "... collected ... twice from residents ... and from one person ... after anthelmintic treatment."

TM: Ingestion of plerocercoid with raw, salted or undercooked fish

Rausch, R. L., Scott, E. M. and Rausch, V. R., 1967, Helminths in Eskimos in Western Alaska, with particular reference to *Diphyllobothrium* infection and anaemia. *Transactions of the Royal Society of Tropical Medicine and Hygiene*, **61**, 351–357.

CYCLOPHYLLIDEA

ANOPLOCEPHALIDAE

Bertiella mucronata (Meyner, 1895) Stiles and Hassall, 1902

DH: MAN; species of non-human primate including *Alouatta caraya* and *A. nigra* (howler monkeys)

IH: Species of oribatid mites

GD: The Americas (Argentina; Brazil; Cuba; Paraguay)

LM: Small intestine; "... eggs and proglottids ... in the feces."

TM: Ingestion of cysticercoid in mite

D'Alessandro, B. A., Beaver, P. C. and Pallares, R. M., 1963, *Bertiella* infection in man in Paraguay. *American Journal of Tropical Medicine and Hygiene*, **12**, 193–198.

Bertiella studeri (Blanchard, 1891) Stiles and Hassall, 1902

DH: MAN; species of non-human primate including *Pongo pygmaeus pygmaeus* (orangutan) and *Macaca radiata* (bonnet monkey)

IH: Species of oribatid mite including *Scheloribates laevigatus*

GD: Africa (Mauritius); Asia (India, Indonesia, Malaysia, Philippines, Singapore, Sri Lanka, Thailand, Yemen)

LM: Small intestine; "... noticed a white object in the faeces on 4–5 occasions ..."

TM: Ingestion of cysticercoid in mite

Bhaibulaya, M., 1985, Human infection with *Bertiella studeri* in Thailand. *Southeast Asian Journal of Tropical Medicine and Public Health*, **16**, 505–507.

Inermicapsifer madagascariensis (Davaine, 1870) Baer, 1956

DH: MAN; species of rodent including *Chinchilla laniger* (*chinchilla*) *and Praomys natalensis* (soft-furred rat)

IH: Presumably species of arthropod

GD: Africa (Comoros Islands, Congo, Kenya, Madagascar, South Africa, Zambia, Zimbabwe); The Americas (Cuba, Venezuela)

LM: Small intestine

TM: Presumably ingestion of cysticercoid in intermediate host

Goldsmid, J. M. and Muir, M., 1972, *Inermicapsifer madagascariensis* (Davaine, 1870) Baer, 1956 (Platyhelminthes: Cestoda) as a parasite of man in Rhodesia. *Central African Journal of Medicine*, **18**, 205–207.

Mathevotaenia symmetrica (Baylis, 1927) Akhumian, 1946

DH: MAN; species of rodent including *Mus musculus* (mouse)

IH: Species of beetle including *Tribolium confusum* (flour beetle) and species of moth including *Plodia interpunctella*

GD: Asia (Thailand); helminth distributed widely in species of rodent

LM: Small intestine; "Detached gravid proglottids ... in the stool ... most closely resembles *M. symmetrica* ..."

TM: Ingestion of cysticercoid in insect

Lamom, C. and Greer, G. J., 1986, Human infection with an anoplocephalid tapeworm of the genus *Mathevotaenia. American Journal of Tropical Medicine and Hygiene*, **35**, 824–826.

Moniezia expansa (Rudolphi, 1805) Blanchard, 1891

DH: MAN; domesticated cattle, goat and sheep and species of herbivorous mammal

IH: Species of oribatid mite including *Galumna virginiensis* and *Scheloribates laevigatus*

GD: Europe (USSR); helminth widely distributed where domesticated ruminant mammals are maintained

LM: Small intestine; "... there were certain symptoms which disappeared on the expulsion of the moniezia." (*Tropical Diseases Bulletin*, **35**, 604)

TM: Ingestion of cysticercoid in oribatid mite

Echov, V. S. and Malyguine, S. A., 1937, Un cas de *Monezia* sp. observe chez l'homme. *Medical Parasitology and Parasitic Diseases, Moscow*, VI, **5**, 627–629.

DAVAINEIDAE

Raillietina (R.) asiatica (von Linstow, 1901) Stiles and Hassall, 1926

DH: MAN

IH: Unresolved

GD: Europe (USSR)

LM: Small intestine; "A single strobila, having about 750 proglottids, was passed by a patient ... eggs ... described ..."

TM: Ingestion of cysticercoid in intermediate host

Beaver, P. C., Jung, R. C. and Cupp, E. W., 1984, *Clinical Parasitology*, 9th edition (Philadelphia: Lea & Febiger) p. 509.

Raillietina (R.) celebensis (Janicki, 1902) Fuhrmann, 1924

DH: MAN; species of rodent including *Mus maeri* (mouse) and *Rattus assimilis* (rat)

IH: Species of ant including *Cardiocondyle nuda*

GD: Asia (China, Japan, Philippines, Taiwan); Oceania (Australia, French Polynesia [Tahiti])

LM: Small intestine; "... eggs and gravid proglottides of ... were recovered in the stools."

TM: Ingestion of cysticercoid in ant

Rougier, Y., Legros, F., Durand, J. P. and Cordoliani, Y., 1981, Four cases of parasitic infection by *Raillietina* (*R.*) *celebensis* (Janicki, 1902) in French Polynesia. *Transactions of the Royal Society of Tropical Medicine and Hygiene*, **75**, 121.

Raillietina (R.) madagascariensis (Davaine, 1869) Fuhrmann, 1924

DH: MAN; species of rodent

IH: Possibly species of cockroach

GD: Asia (Indonesia, Thailand)

LM: Small intestine; "... worms were found in the stools ... two worms were found complete ..."

TM: Ingestion of cysticercoid in intermediate host

Margono, S. S., Handojo, I., Hadidjaja, P. and Mahfudin, H., 1977, *Raillietina* infection in children in Indonesia. *Southeast Asian Journal of Tropical Medicine and Public Health*, **8**, 195–199.

DILEPIDIDAE

Dipylidium caninum (Linnaeus, 1758) Leuckart, 1863

DH: MAN; domesticated cat and dog, species of carnivorous mammal

IH: Species of flea including *Ctenocephalis canis, C. felis* and *Pulex irritans*

GD: Africa (Zimbabwe); The Americas (Argentina; Brazil; Chile; Mexico; USA, Louisiana); Asia (China, Japan, Philippines); The Caribbean (Puerto Rico); Europe (Italy, Portugal, U.K.); Oceania (Australia)

LM: Small intestine

ND: Dipylidiasis due to *Dipylidium caninum*

TM: Ingestion of cysticercoid in flea

Shane, S. M., Adams, R. C., Miller, J. E., Smith, R. E. and Thompson, A. K., 1986, A case of *Dipylidium caninum* in Baton Rouge, Louisiana. *International Journal of Zoonoses*, **13**, 59–62.

HYMENOLEPIDIDAE

Drepanidotaenia lanceolata (Bloch, 1782) Railliet, 1892

DH: MAN; species of anseriform bird (ducks, geese and swans)

IH: Several species of copepod including *Cyclops viridis* and *Diaptomus gracilis*

GD: Helminth distributed worldwide in anseriform birds

LM: Presumably small intestine

TM: Ingestion of cysticercoid in copepod

McDonald, M. E., 1969, *Catalogue of Helminths of Waterfowl (Anatidae)*. (Washington D.C.: U.S. Department of the Interior, Bureau of Sport Fisheries and Wildlife) p. 482.

Hymenolepis diminuta (Rudolphi, 1819) Weinland, 1858

DH: MAN; species of rodent including rat, mouse and *Praomys tullbergi jacksoni* (soft-furred rat)

IH: Species of arthropod including *Tinea granilla* (moth), *Anisolabis arnulipes* (earwig), *Ctenocephalides canis* (flea), *Fontaria virginiensis* (myriapod), *Tenebrio molitor*, *Tribolium castaneum* and *T. confusum* (beetles)

GD: Africa; Asia (China, India, Japan, Philippines); The Americas (Argentina, Brazil, Colombia, Cuba, Equador, Nicaragua, Venezuela); The Caribbean (Granada, Martinique); Europe (Belgium, Italy, USSR); helminth distributed worldwide in rodents

LM: Small intestine

ND: Hymenolepiasis due to *Hymenolepis diminuta*

TM: Ingestion of cysticercoid in arthropod

Edelman, M. H., Springarn, C. L., Nauenbelg, W. G. and Gregory, C., 1965, *Hymenolepis diminuta* (rat tapeworm) infection in man. *American Journal of Medicine*, **38**, 951–953.

Vampirolepis nana (Siebold, 1852) Spasskii, 1954

S: *Hymenolepis nana*

DH: MAN; worm may also infect species of rodent

GD: Worldwide (more common in warm than in cool climates)

LM: Small intestine

ND: Hymenolepiasis due to *Hymenolepis nana*

TM: Ingestion of egg leads to development of cysticercoid in intestinal mucosa subsequently giving rise to adult tapeworm. Some authorities point out that *V. nana* may also develop to the cysticercoid in an intermediate host (*Ctenocephalides canis* [flea] and *Tenebrio molitor* [beetle]) in which case humans could become infected on ingestion of insects carrying cysticercoids.

Sahbra, G. H., Arfaa, F. and Bijan, H., 1967, Intestinal helminthiases in the rural area of Khuzestan, South-west Iran. *Annals of Tropical Medicine and Parasitology*, **61**, 352–357.

MESOCESTOIDAE

Mesocestoides lineatus (Goeze, 1782) Railliet, 1893

DH: MAN; many species of carnivorous mammal

IH1: Possibly species of arthropod

IH2: Species of amphibian, reptile and small mammalian species

GD: Asia (China, Japan, Korea)

LM: Small intestine

TM: Presumably ingestion of tetrathyridium (modified cysticercoid) with raw or undercooked second intermediate host

Kagei, N., Kihata, M., Shimizu, S., Urabe, M. and Ishii, A., 1974, The 10th case of human infection with *Mesocestoides lineatus* (Cestoda: Cyclophyllidea) in Japan. *Japanese Journal of Parasitology*, **23**, 380–382.

Mesocestoides variabilis Mueller, 1927

DH: MAN; many species of carnivorous mammal

IH1: Unresolved

IH2: Species of wild and domestic bird, snake, frog and rodent

GD: The Americas (Greenland; USA, Missouri, Texas)

LM: Small intestine; "child ... treated with atebrine ... contained individual proglottids and strobilae ..."

TM: Presumably ingestion of tetrathyridium (modified cysticercoid) with raw or undercooked second intermediate host

Gleason, N. N. and Healy, G. R., 1967, Report of a case of *Mesocestoides* (Cestoda) in a child in Missouri. *Journal of Parasitology*, **53**, 83–84.

TAENIIDAE

Echinococcus granulosus (Batsch, 1786) Rudolphi, 1810

DH: Dog and various species of carnivorous mammal

IH: MAN; many species of mammal including domesticated ungulates and wild herbivores

GD: Worldwide, particularly in sheep and cattle rearing countries

LM: Hydatid cyst found in liver, lungs, bone cavities, brain and other sites

ND: Echinococcosis due to *Echinococcus granulosus*

TM: Ingestion of egg in contaminated food or herbage

Smyth, J. D., 1987, Changing concepts in the microecology, macroecology and epidemiology of hydatid disease. In *Helminth Zoonoses*, edited by S. Geerts, V. Kumar and G. D. Brandt. (Dordrecht, Boston, Lancaster: Martinus Nijhoff), pp. 3–11.

Echinococcus multilocularis (Leuckart, 1863) Vogel, 1955

DH: Dog and other species of carnivore including *Alopex lagopus* (arctic fox) and *Vulpes vulpes* (red fox)

IH: MAN; species of rodent including *Microtus oeconomus* (tundra vole) and *Peromyscus maniculatus* (deer mouse)

GD: The Americas (Argentina; Canada; Uruguay; USA, Alaska, Minnesota); Asia (China, Japan, Turkey); Europe (France, Iceland, Italy, Poland, USSR)

LM: Multilocular cyst in liver with secondary cysts in other organs

ND: Echinococcosis due to *Echinococcus multilocularis*

TM: Ingestion of egg in contaminated food or herbage

Muller, R., 1975, *Worms and Disease* (London: William Heinemann Medical Books Ltd.), pp. 57–59.

Echinococcus oligarthrus (Diesing, 1863) Lühe, 1910

DH: Species of wild felids including *Felis concolor* (puma), *Felis onca* (jaguar) and *Felis yagouaroundi* (wild cat)

IH: MAN; species of small mammal including *Cuniculus paca* (paca), *Didelphis marsupialis* (opossum) and *Sylvilagus floridanus* (wild rabbit)

GD: The Americas (Venezuela)

LM: "... single cyst localized intraorbitally and behind the left eye retroocular."

ND: Echinococcosis due to *Echinococcus oligarthrus*

TM: Ingestion of egg in contaminated food or herbage

Lopera, R. D., Melendez, R. D., Fernandez, I., Spirit, J. and Perera, M. P., 1989, Orbital hydatid cyst of *Echinococcus oligarthrus* in a human in Venezuela. *Journal of Parasitology*, **75**, 467–470.

Echinococcus vogeli Rausch and Bernstein, 1972

DH: Domesticated dog and *Speothos venaticus* (bush dog)

IH: MAN; *Cuniculus paca* (paca)

GD: The Americas (Colombia, Costa Rica, Ecuador, Panama, Venezuela)

LM: "... tumor-like mass in or near the liver ... intercostal space ... were in the chest."

ND: Echinococcosis due to *Echinococcus vogeli*

TM: Ingestion of egg in contaminated food or herbage

D'Alessandro, A., Rausch, R. L., Cuello, C. and Aristizabal, N., 1979, *Echinococcus vogeli* in man with a review on polycystic hydatid disease in Colombia and neighbouring countries. *American Journal of Tropical Medicine and Hygiene*, **28**, 303–317.

Multiceps brauni (Setti, 1897)

DH: Domesticated dog, *Canis mesomelas* (black-backed jackal) and *Lycaon pictus* (African wild dog)

IH: MAN; various species of rodent

GD: Africa (Uganda)

LM: Eye and orbit (anterior chamber, subconjunctival, vitreous); "... all the cases seen in Uganda conform to a type and most closely resemble the species named *brauni* ..."

ND: Coenurosis due to *Multiceps brauni*

TM: Presumably ingestion of egg in contaminated food or herbage

Williams, P. H. and Templeton, A. C., 1971, Infection of the eye by the tapeworm *Coenurus. British Journal of Ophthamology*, **55**, 766–769.

Multiceps glomeratus (Railliet and Henry, 1915) Brumpt 1922

DH: Unresolved

IH: MAN; species of rodent including *Gerbillus pyramidum* (gerbil)

GD: Africa (Nigeria)

LM: "... a cystic tapeworm ... in a tumour ... excised from an intercostal muscle."

ND: Coenurosis due to *Multiceps glomeratus*

TM: Ingestion of egg in contaminated food or herbage

Turner, M. and Leiper, R. T., 1919, On the occurrence of *Coenurus glomeratus* in man in West Africa. *Transactions of the Royal Society of Tropical Medicine and Hygiene*, **13**, 23–24.

Multiceps longihamatus (Morishita and Sawada, 1966)

DH: MAN

IH: Possibly rabbit and hare

GD: Asia (Japan)

LM: Small intestine; "... three tapeworms ... passed with ... stool."

TM: Ingestion of coenurus with raw or undercooked intermediate host

Morishita, K. and Sawada, I., 1966, On tapeworms of the genus *Multiceps* hitherto unrecorded from man. *Japanese Journal of Parasitology*, **15**, 495–501.

Multiceps multiceps Leske, 1780

DH: Domesticated dog, species of carnivorous mammal including *Canis lupus* (wolf) and *Alopex lagopus* (Arctic fox)

IH: MAN; species of herbivorous mammal and species of non-human primate including *Macaca mulatta* (rhesus monkey) and *M. silenus* (lion tailed macaque)

GD: Africa (South Africa, Uganda); The Americas (Brazil; USA, South Dakota); Europe (U.K., France)

LM: "A suboccipital craniotomy ... exposed a multiloculated cyst ..."

ND: Coenurosis due to *Multiceps multiceps*

TM: Ingestion of egg with contaminated food or herbage

Hermos, J. A., Healy, G. R., Schultz, M. G., Barlow, J. and Church, W. G., 1970, Fatal human cerebral coenurosis. *Journal of the American Medical Association*, **213**, 1461–1464.

Multiceps serialis (Gervais, 1847) Baillet, 1863

DH: Domesticated dog and species of carnivore including *Canis lupus* (wolf) and *Hyaena hyaena* (hyena)

IH: MAN; rabbit, hare and species of rodent

GD: The Americas (Canada, USA)

LM: "... of a hemorrhagic mass in the left breast led to the surgical removal of bladder-like cysts ... identified as larvae of *Taenia serialis*."

ND: Coenurosis due to *Multiceps serialis*

TM: Ingestion of egg with contaminated food or herbage

Benger, A., Rennie, R. P., Roberts, T., Thornley, J. H. and Scholten, T., 1981, A human coenurus infection in Canada. *American Journal of Tropical Medicine and Hygiene*, **30**, 638–644.

Taenia crassiceps (Zeder, 1800) Rudolphi, 1810

DH: Domesticated dog; species of carnivorous mammal including *Felix lynx* (lynx) and *Vulpes vulpes* (fox)

IH: MAN; species of rodent

GD: The Americas (Canada, Ontario; USA); helminth distributed worldwide in mammal hosts

LM: "... A cysticercus of *Taenia crassiceps* ... was removed from between the retina and retinal pigment epithelium of a ... (patient) ..."

TM: Ingestion of egg with contaminated food or herbage

Freeman, R. S., Fallis, A. M., Shea, M., Maberley, A. I. and Walters, J., 1973, Intraocular *Taenia crassiceps* (Cestoda) part II. The parasite. *American Journal of Tropical Medicine and Hygiene*, **22**, 493–495.

Taenia solium Linnaeus, 1758

DH: MAN; experimentally in *Hylobates lar* (lar gibbon)

IH: MAN; domesticated pig

GD: Worldwide where humans and pigs are associated

LM: Adult worm located in intestine, cysticercus larva in brain (neurocysticercosis) and subcutaneous tissue

ND: Taeniasis due to *Taenia solium* (adult, when human is DH)
Cysticercosis due to *Taenia solium* (larva, when human is IH)

TM: Ingestion of cysticercus with raw or undercooked pork (DH) or ingestion of egg (IH)

Cruz, M., Davis, A., Dixon, H., Pawlowski, Z. S. and Proano, J., 1989, Operational studies on the control of *Taenia solium* taeniasis/cysticercosis in Ecuador. *Bulletin of the World Health Organization*, **67**, 401–407.

Taenia taeniaeformis (Batsch, 1796)

DH: Domesticated cat and dog, species of carnivore including *Mustela foina* (weasel)

IH: MAN; species of rodent

GD: The Americas (Argentina); Europe (Czechoslovakia)

LM: Liver

TM: Ingestion of egg with contaminated food or herbage

Sterba, J. and Barus, V., 1976, First record of *Strobilocercus fasciolaris* (Taeniidae-larvae) in man. *Folia Parasitologia*, **23**, 221–226.

Taeniarhynchus saginatus (Goeze, 1782) Weinland, 1858

S: *Taenia saginata*

DH: MAN

IH: Many species of herbivorous mammal including domesticated cattle and *Rangifer rangifer* (reindeer)

GD: Worldwide where humans and cattle are associated

LM: Adult worm located in small intestine, occasionally other sites; cysticerci, identified as *T. saginatus*, have been found in human tissue

ND: Taeniasis due to *Taenia saginata*

TM: Ingestion of cysticercus with raw or undercooked beef

Pawlowski, Z. S. and Schultz, M. G., 1972, Taeniasis and cysticercosis (*Taenia saginata*). *Advances in Parasitology*, **10**, 269–343.

NEMATODA

DIOCTOPHYMATIDAE

Dioctophyma renale (Goeze, 1782) Stiles, 1901

DH: MAN; various species of mammal including domesticated dog and horse, rat, *Lutra lutra* (otter), *Mustela vison* (mink), *Procyon lotor* (raccoon) and *Vulpes vulpes* (fox)

IH: Species of aquatic oligochaete including *Cambarincola philadelphica* (N. America) and *Lumbricus variegatus* (USSR)

PH: *Ameiurus melas* (bullhead); other species of freshwater fish and frogs

GD: The Americas (Canada, USA); Asia (Iran, Southeast Asia); Europe (USSR)

LM: Kidney

ND: Pyelonephritis due to *Dioctophyme renalis*

TM: Ingestion of infective larva in raw or undercooked fish and frogs

Beaver, P. C. and Theis, J. H., 1979, Dioctophymatid larval nematode in a subcutaneous nodule from man in California. *American Journal of Tropical Medicine and Hygiene*, **28**, 20–21.

Eustrongylides sp.

DH: MAN; species of piscivorous bird including *Ardea herodias* (great blue heron)

IH1: Species of aquatic oligochaete

IH2: Species of freshwater fish including *Fundulus heteroclitus* (killifish)

GD: The Americas (USA, Maryland)

LM: "Laparotomy showed in one patient two nematodes in the abdominal cavity, the other penetrating the caecal wall."

TM: Ingestion of infective larva in raw or undercooked fish

Guerin, P. F. S., Marapendi, S., McGrail, L., Moravec, C. L. and Schiller, E. L., 1982, Intestinal perforation caused by larval *Eustrongylides*—Maryland. *Centers for Disease Control, Morbidity and Mortality Weekly Reports*, **31**, 383–389.

TRICHINELLIDAE

Trichinella nativa

DH/IH: MAN; various species of mammal including *Thalarotos maritimus* (polar bear) and *Odobenus rosmarus* (walrus)

GD: The Americas (Greenland; USA, Alaska); helminth distributed in arctic and sub-arctic regions

LM: Presumably adult worm associated with intestinal mucosa; larva encysted in striated muscle

TM: Presumably ingestion of infective larva in raw or undercooked fish

Pozio, E., La Rosa, G. and Rossi, P., 1989, *Trichinella* Reference Centre. *Parasitology Today*, **5**, 169–170.

Trichinella nelsoni Britov and Boev, 1972

DH/IH: MAN, various species of mammal including domesticated dog, horse, pig and *Canis lupus* (wolf) and *Vulpes vulpes* (fox)

GD: Europe (France, Italy)

LM: Adult worm associated with intestinal mucosa; larva encysted in striated muscle

TM: Ingestion of infective larva in raw or undercooked meat

Pozio, E., Cappelli, O., Marchesi, L., Valeri, P. and Rossi, P., 1988, Third outbreak of trichinellosis caused by consumption of horse meat in Italy. *Annales de Parasitologie Humaine et Comparee*, **63**, 48–53.

Trichinella spiralis (Owen, 1835) Railliet, 1896

DH/IH: MAN; domesticated cat and dog, many species of mammal including bear, mouse, pig, rat and *Procyon lotor* (raccoon)

GD: Worldwide

LM: Adult worm associated with intestinal mucosa; larva encysted in striated muscle

ND: Trichinellosis

TM: Ingestion of infective (encysted) larva in raw or undercooked meat especially pork

Steele, J. H., 1982, Trichinosis. In *CRC Handbook Series in Zoonoses. Section C. Parasitic Zoonoses*, Volume II, edited by M. G. Schultz, (Boca Raton, Florida: CRC Press, Inc.), pp. 293–326.

TRICHURIDAE

Anatrichosoma cutaneum (Swift, Boots and Miles, 1922) Chitwood and Smith, 1956

DH: MAN; *Macaca mulatta* (rhesus monkey)

IH: Unresolved

GD: Asia (Japan, Vietnam); helminth found in monkeys in Africa and Asia

LM: "Skin lesions ... dug into the epidermis."

TM: Presumably through skin penetration by an infective larva from contaminated soil

Le-Van-Hoa, Duong-Hong-Mo and Nguyen-Lun-Vien, 1963, Premier cas de capillariose cutanee humaine. *Bulletin de la Societe de Pathologie Exotique*, **56**, 121–126.

Aonchotheca philippinensis (Chitwood, Velasquez and Salazar, 1968) Moravec, 1982

S: *Capillaria philippinensis*

DH: MAN; experimentally in gerbil, monkey and rat; species of bird considered potential natural hosts

IH: *Hypseleotris bibartita* (bagsit); experimentally in other species of brackish water and freshwater fish

GD: Africa (Egypt); Asia (Iran, Japan, Philippines, Thailand)

LM: Small intestine, mainly jejunum

ND: Intestinal capillariasis

TM: Probably by ingestion of infective larva in raw or undercooked fish

Cross, J. H., 1990, Intestinal capillariasis. *Parasitology Today*, **6**, 26–28.

Calodium hepaticum (Bancroft, 1893) Moravec, 1982

S: *Capillaria hepatica*

DH: MAN; rat and many species of mammal

GD: Africa (South Africa); The Americas (Brazil, Mexico, USA); Asia (India, Turkey); Europe (Czechoslovakia, Italy)

LM: Liver

ND: Hepatic capillariasis

TM: Ingestion of infective egg, containing first-stage larva, presumably from contaminated soil

Attah, E., Nagarajan, S., Obineche, E. and Gera, S., 1983, Hepatic capillariasis. *American Journal of Clinical Pathology*, **79**, 127–130.

Eucoleus aerophilus (Creplin, 1839) Dujardin, 1845

S: *Capillaria aerophila*

DH: MAN; domesticated cat and dog, *Vulpes vulpes* (fox) and other species of carnivorous mammal

GD: Africa (Morocco); Asia (Iran); Europe (USSR); helminth also found in animal hosts in The Americas and Oceania

LM: Respiratory tract

ND: Pulmonary capillariasis due to *Capillaria aerophila*

TM: Ingestion of egg containing infective larva, presumably from contaminated soil

Aftandelians, R., Raafat, F., Taffozoli, M. and Beaver, P. C., 1977, Pulmonary capillariasis in a child in Iran. *American Journal of Tropical Medicine and Hygiene*, **26**, 64–71.

Trichuris suis Schrank, 1788

DH: Man; domesticated pig

GD: Helminth widely distributed in countries with temperate climate where pigs are reared

LM: Large intestine; "... been reported rarely from the human intestine."

TM: Ingestion of infective egg, presumably from contaminated soil

Barriga, O. O., 1982, Trichuriasis. In *CRC Handbook Series in Zoonoses. Section C: Parasitic Zoonoses*, Volume II, edited by M. G. Schultz, (Boca Raton, Florida: CRC Press Inc.), pp. 339–345.

Trichuris trichiura (Linnaeus, 1771) Stiles, 1901

DH: MAN; various species of non-human primate

GD: Worldwide

LM: Associated with the mucosa of the large intestine, particularly the colon

ND: Trichuriasis

TM: Ingestion of egg containing infective larva from contaminated soil

Bundy, D. A. P. and Cooper, E. S., 1989, *Trichuris* and trichuriasis in humans. *Advances in Parasitology*, **28**, 108–173.

Trichuris vulpis (Froelich, 1789)

DH: MAN; domesticated dog and species of canine mammal

GD: The Americas (USA); The Caribbean (Bahamas); Europe (Italy); helminth distributed in dogs worldwide

LM: "... gravid female ... was found in histopathologic sections of an appendix ..."

TM: Presumably ingestion of egg containing infective larva from contaminated soil

Kenney, M. and Eveland, L. R., 1978, Infection of man with *Trichuris vulpis*, the whipworm of dogs. *American Journal of Clinical Pathology*, **69**, 199.

MERMITHIDAE

Agamomermis hominis oris (Leidy, 1852)

H: Man; free-living adult worm in soil after development in body of grasshopper

GD: Helminth widely distributed

LM: Presumably small intestine; "... a nematode ... collected from the faeces ... of a five-year-old girl."

TM: Presumably, accidental ingestion of larva in insect or of free-living worm from soil

Poinar, G. O., 1979, *Nematodes for Biological Control of Insects*, (Boca Raton, Florida: CRC Press Inc.), pp. 225–231.

Agamomermis restiformis (Leidy, 1880)

H: Man; free-living adult worm in soil after development in body of grasshopper

GD: Helminth widely distributed

LM: "... removed from the urethra of a man in the United States."

TM: Presumably, accidental ingestion of larva in insect or of free-living worm from soil

Poinar, G. O., 1979, *Nematodes for Biological Contol of Insects*, (Boca Raton, Florida: CRC Press Inc.), pp. 225-231.

Mermis nigrescens Dujardin, 1842

H: Man; free-living adult worm in soil after development in body cavity of grasshopper

GD: Helminth widely distributed

LM: "... a nematode (gravid female) was removed from the mouth of a 1-month-old infant ..."

TM: Presumably accidental ingestion of worm from contaminated vegetation

Poinar, G. O. and Hoberg, E. P., 1988, *Mermis nigrescens* (Mermithidae: Nematoda) recovered from the mouth of a child. *American Journal of Tropical Medicine and Hygiene*, **39**, 478-479.

CEPHALOBIDAE

Micronema deletrix Anderson and Bemrick, 1965

H: Man; free-living species of saprophagous nematode in soil

GD: The Americas (Canada; USA, Texas, Washington D.C.)

LM: "... died of a meningoencephalitis ... *Micronema* were in the brain, liver and heart."

ND: Meningoencephalitis due to *Micronema deletrix*

TM: Invasion of body through deep lacerations

Gardiner, C. H., Koh, D. S. and Cardella, T. A., 1981, *Micronema* in man: third fatal infection. *American Journal of Tropical Medicine and Hygiene,* **30,** 586–589.

Turbatrix aceti (Müller, 1783) Peters, 1927

H: Man; free-living species of microbivorous nematode in vinegar

GD: The Americas (Mexico)

LM: "... a specimen was taken with a catheter ... numerous worms of all stages were found"

TM: Possibly accidental introduction of worms into ureter or vagina when contaminated vinegar is used as a douche

Stiles, C. W. and Frankland, W. A., 1902, A case of vinegar eel infection in the human bladder. *Bureau of Animal Industry Bulletin,* **35,** 35–40.

RHABDITIDAE

Cheilobus quadrilabiatus Cobb, 1924

H: Man; free-living species of saprophagous nematode in soil

GD: Europe (South-east Czechoslovakia)

LM: Presumably alimentary tract; "... in the faeces of pupils from Southern region of Slovakia ..."

TM: Unresolved

Dziuban, M., 1967, On the specificity of some species of the suborder Rhabditida. *Helminthologia,* **8,** 121–125.

Diploscapter coronata Cobb, 1913

H: Man; free-living species of saprophagous nematode in soil

GD: The Americas (USA, Texas)

LM: "... was found, apparently established and multiplying, in stomachs which entirely lacked, or had reduced amounts of, hydrochloric acid."

TM: Accidental ingestion of worms associated with vegetation

Chandler, A. C., 1938, *Diploscapter coronata* as a facultative parasite of man, with a general review of vertebrate parasitism by rhabditoid worms. *Parasitology*, **30**, 44–45.

Pelodera strongyloides (Schneider, 1860) Schneider, 1866

H: Man; free-living species of saprophagous nematode in soil. Also occasionally found in rodents and various species of domesticated mammal

GD: Europe (Poland)

LM: "... cultures were set up, from larvae found in the child's skin ... showed typical features of *Rhabditis strongyloides* ..."

TM: Presumably worms in soil enter skin

Pasyk, K., 1978, *Dermatitis rhabditidosa* in an 11-year-old girl. A cutaneous parasitic disease of man. *British Journal of Dermatology*, **98**, 107–112.

Pelodera teres Schneider, 1866

S: *Rhabditis donbass*

H: Man; free-living species of saprophagous nematode in soil

LM: Presumably alimentary tract, worms observed to develop in human faeces having presumably gained access as a contaminator of food or drink

TM: Accidental ingestion of worms in contaminated food

Beaver, P. C., Jung, R. C. and Cupp, E. W., 1984, *Clinical Parasitology*, 9th edition (Philadelphia: Lea & Febiger). (See p. 263).

Rhabditis axei (Cobbold, 1884)

H: Man; free-living species of saprophagous nematode in soil

GD: Africa (Zimbabwe); Asia (China)

LM: "a urine specimen ... from an African female ... was found to contain
         ova, living larvae and living males and females of what appeared to be
         Rhabditis (Rhabditella) axei".

TM: Unresolved

Goldsmid, J. M., 1967, *Rhabditis (Rhabditella) axei* in the urine of an African in Rhodesia.
Journal of Helminthology, **41**, 305–308.

Rhabditis elongata Schneider, 1866

H: Man; free-living species of saprophagous nematode in soil

GD: Asia (South Korea)

LM: Presumably alimentary tract; "... result of a faecal examination ...
         found 2 cases ... in 16-year-old high school girls".

TM: Unresolved

Lee, W. K., Choi, W. C. and Lee, O. R., 1978, *Rhabditis elongata* Schneider, 1866 from
students in Korea. *Korean Journal of Parasitology*, **16**, 113–116.

Rhabditis inermis (Schneider, 1866) Dougherty, 1955

S: *Rhabditis hominis; R. faecalis; R. schachtiella*

H: Man; free-living saprophagous nematode in soil

GD: Asia (Japan)

LM: Presumably alimentary tract; "... all stages of development ... found numerously in freshly passed faeces ..." in 17 out of 668 school children

TM: Presumably accidental ingestion of worms associated with vegetation

Kobayashi, H., 1920, On a new species of rhabditoid worms found in the human intestine. *Journal of Parasitology*, **6**, 148–151.

Rhabditis niellyi Blanchard, 1855

H: Man; free-living species of saprophagous nematode in soil

GD: Europe (France)

LM: Skin

TM: Unresolved

Nielly, M., 1882, Un cas de dermatose parasitaire non encore observee en France (*Anguillula leptodera*). *Bulletin de L'Academie Nationale de Medecine, Paris*, **46**, 395–402.

Rhabditis pellio (Schneider, 1866) Bütschli, 1873

H: Man; free-living species of saprophagous nematode in soil

GD: The Americas (Mexico)

LM: Vagina; "... numerous specimens in different stages of development"

TM: Unresolved

Cabellero, y. C. E., 1937, Un caso de parasitismo accidental por *Rhabditis pellio* en Mexico. *Annales del Instituto de Biologia, Mexico*, **8**, 393–395.

Rhabditis taurica Mireckij and Skrajabin, 1965

H: Man; free-living species of saprophagous nematode in soil

GD: Europe (USSR, Simferopol)

LM: Presumably alimentary tract; "... in the faeces of a 6-year-old child ..."

TM: Unresolved

Mireckij, D. J. and Skrajabin, A. S., 1965, Discovery of *Rhabditis taurica* sp. nov. in a child. *Helminthologia*, **6**, 13–16.

Rhabditis terricola Dujardin, 1845

H: Man; free-living species of saprophagous nematode in soil

GD: Europe (South-east Czechoslovakia)

LM: Presumably alimentary tract; "... in the faeces of pupils from the Southern regions of Slovakia ..."

TM: Unresolved

Dziuban, M., 1967, On the specificity of some species of the suborder Rhabditata. *Helminthologia*, **8**, 121–125.

Rhabditis sp. Dujardin, 1845

H: Man; free-living saprophagous nematode in soil

GD: Asia (South Korea)

LM: Presumably alimentary tract; "Five cases infected ... detected in ... stool specimens from rural primary school children. The five cases were re-examined ... *Rhabditis* sp. were detected again in 4 cases."

TM: Unresolved

Ahn, Y. K., Chung, P. R. and Lee, K. T., 1985, *Rhabditis* sp. infected cases in rural school children. *Korean Journal of Parasitology*, **23**, 1–6.

STRONGYLOIDIDAE

Strongyloides canis Brumpt, 1922

DH: Man (experimental)

GD: Helminth distributed in Europe

LM: Larval stage in skin

TM: Presumably skin penetration by infective third-stage larva

Augustine, D. L., 1940, Experimental studies on the validity of species in the genus *Strongyloides*. *American Journal of Hygiene*, **32**, 24–32.

Strongyloides cebus Darling, 1911

DH: Man (experimental); *Cebus capucinus* (white-throated capucin). *Strongyloides cebus* has a free-living (heterogonic) cycle and a parasitic (homogonic) cycle

GD: The Americas (Panama)

LM: Larval stage in skin

TM: Skin penetration by infective third-stage larva

Sandground, J. H., 1925, Speciation and specificity in the nematode genus *Strongyloides*. *Journal of Parasitology*, **12**, 59–81.

Strongyloides felis (Chandler, 1925)

DH: Man (experimental); domesticated cat. *Strongyloides felis* has a free-living (heterogonic) cycle and a parasitic (homogonic) cycle

GD: Oceania (Australia)

LM: Larval stage in skin

TM: Skin penetration by infective third-stage larva

Speare, R., 1989, Identification of species of *Strongyloides*. In: *Strongyloidiasis a Major Roundworm Infection of Man*, edited by D. I. Grove, (London: Taylor & Francis), pp. 11–83.

Strongyloides fuelleborni von Linstow, 1905

DH: MAN; various species of non-human primate. *Strongyloides fuelleborni* has a free-living (heterogonic) cycle and a parasitic (homogonic) cycle

GD: Africa (Ethiopia, Malawi, Namibia, Rwanda, Zambia, Zimbabwe)

LM: Adult parthenogenetic female in mucosa of small intestine, larva migrates through skin and tissues

ND: Strongyloidiasis due to *Strongyloides fuelleborni*

TM: Skin penetration by infective third-stage larva, transmammary transmission

Ashford, R. W. and Barnish, G., 1989, *Strongyloides fuelleborni* and similar parasites in animals and man. In *Strongyloidiasis a Major Roundworm Infection of Man*, edited by D. I. Grove, (London and Philadelphia: Taylor & Francis), pp. 271–286.

Strongyloides cf *fuelleborni* (taxonomy unresolved)

DH: MAN; *Strongyloides* cf *fuelleborni* has a free-living (heterogonic) cycle and a parasitic (homogonic) cycle

GD: Oceania (Papua New Guinea)

LM: Adult parthenogenetic female in mucosa of small intestine, presumably larva migrates through skin and tissues

TM: Unresolved, presumably skin penetration by infective third-stage larva, transmammary route suspected

Ashford, R. W. and Barnish, G., 1989, *Strongyloides fuelleborni* and similar parasites in animals and man. In *Strongyloidiasis a Major Roundworm Infection of Man*, edited by D. I. Grove, (London and Philadelphia: Taylor & Francis), pp. 271–286.

Strongyloides myopotami Artigas and Pacheco, 1933

DH: Man (experimental); *Myocastor coypus* (nutria), *Myopotamis coypus* (coipu rat) and *Procyon lotor* (raccoon). *Strongyloides myopotami* has a free-living (heterogonic) cycle and a parasitic (homogonic) cycle

GD: The Americas (Brazil)

LM: Larval stage in skin

TM: Skin penetration by infective third-stage larva

Little, M. D., 1965, Dermatitis in a human volunteer infected with *Strongyloides* of nutria and raccoon. *American Journal of Tropical Medicine and Hygiene*, **14**, 1007–1009.

Strongyloides papillosus (Wedl, 1856) Ransom, 1911

DH: Man; domesticated sheep and goat and various species of wild and domesticated mammal. *Strongyloides papillosus* has a free-living (heterogonic) cycle and a parasitic (homogonic) cycle

GD: Helminth widely distributed in animal hosts

LM: "... skin penetration of the hands ... by larvae of *Strongyloides papillosus* ..."

TM: Presumably skin penetration by infective third-stage larva

Roeckel, I. E. and Lyons, E. T., 1977, Cutaneous larva migrans, an occupational disease. *Annals of Clinical Laboratory Science*, **7**, 405–410.

Strongyloides planiceps Rogers, 1943

DH: Man (experimental); domesticated cat and dog, *Felis planiceps* (flat-headed cat) and *Vulpes vulpes* (fox). *Strongyloides planiceps* has a free-living (heterogonic) cycle and a parasitic (homogonic) cycle

GD: Asia (Japan)

LM: Larval stage in skin

TM: Skin penetration by infective third-stage larva

Miyamoto, K., 1986, The prevalence of strongyloidiasis in stray dogs, cats and red foxes of Hokkaido and the resistance of eggs and filariform larvae of *Strongyloides planiceps* to various environmental factors. *Japanese Journal of Parasitology*, **35**, 512–520.

Strongyloides procyonis Little, 1965

DH: MAN (experimental); *Procyon lotor* (raccoon). *Strongyloides procyonis* has a free-living (heterogonic) cycle and a parasitic (homogonic) cycle

GD: The Americas (USA, Louisiana)

LM: Presumably, adult parthenogenetic female in mucosa of small intestine, larva migrates through skin and tissues

TM: Skin penetration by infective third-stage larva

Little, M. D., 1965, Dermatitis in a human volunteer infected with *Strongyloides* of nutria and raccoon. *American Journal of Tropical Medicine and Hygiene*, **14**, 1007–1009.

Strongyloides ransomi Schwartz and Alicata, 1930

DH: Man; domesticated pig and rabbit. *Strongyloides ransomi* has a free-living (heterogonic) cycle and a parasitic (homogonic) cycle

GD: Helminth widely distributed in domesticated pigs

LM: "... skin penetration of the hands ... by larvae of *Strongyloides ransomi* ..."

TM: Presumably skin penetration by infective third-stage larva (prenatal and transmammary transmission in pig)

Roeckel, I. E. and Lyons, E. T., 1977, Cutaneous larva migrans, an occupational disease. *Annals of Clinical and Laboratory Science*, **7**, 405–410.

Strongyloides simiae Hung, see Lu and Hoeppli, 1923

DH: Man (experimental); various species of non-human primate. *Strongyloides simiae* has a free-living (heterogonic) cycle and a parasitic (homogonic) cycle

GD: Africa (Guinea-Bissau)

LM: Larval stage in skin

TM: Skin penetration by infective third-stage larva

de Azevedo, J. F. and de Meira, M. T. V., 1946, Helminas intestinaise de macacos de Guine Portuguesa. Tentativa de infestacao experimental do homen et animais com o *Strongyloides simiae*. *Anais do Institut de Medicana Tropical*, **3**, 267–276.

Strongyloides stercoralis (Bavay, 1876) Stiles and Hassall, 1902

DH: MAN; domesticated cat and dog, various species of non-human primate. *Strongyloides stercoralis* has a free-living (heterogonic) cycle and a parasitic (homogonic) cycle

GD: Worldwide

LM: Adult parthenogenetic female in the mucosa of the small intestine, larva migrates through skin and tissues

ND: Strongyloidiasis due to *Strongyloides stercoralis*

TM: Skin penetration by infective third-stage larva, autoinfection by larva released in small intestine

Grove, D. I. (editor), 1989, *Strongyloidiasis a Major Roundworm Infection of Man.* (London and Philadelphia: Taylor & Francis).

Strongyloides westeri Ihle, 1917

DH: Man; domesticated horse and pig, guinea-pig, mouse, rabbit. *Strongyloides westeri* has a free-living (heterogonic) cycle and a parasitic (homogonic) cycle

GD: Helminth widely distributed in animal hosts

LM: "... skin penetration of the hands ... by larvae of *Strongyloides westeri* ..."

TM: Presumably skin penetration by infective third-stage larva

Roeckel, I. E. and Lyons, E. T., 1977, Cutaneous larva migrans, an occupational disease. *Annals of Clinical Laboratory Science*, **7**, 405–410.

ANCYLOSTOMATIDAE

Ancylostoma braziliense de Faria, 1910

DH: Man; various species of domesticated and wild canine and feline mammals

GD: The Americas (Argentina, Brazil, Uruguay, USA); Africa (South Africa); Asia (India, Philippines); Europe (France, Spain); Oceania (Australia). (Some localities doubtful due to problems of identification.)

LM: Larval stage in skin

ND: Cutaneous larva migrans due to *Ancylostoma braziliense*

TM: Skin penetration by or ingestion of infective third-stage larva

Yoshida, Y., Kondo, K., Kurimoto, H., Fukutome, S. and Shirasaka, S., 1974, Comparative studies on *Ancylostoma braziliense* and *Ancylostoma ceylanicum*. III. Life history in the definitive host. *Journal of Parasitology*, **60**, 636–641.

Ancylostoma caninum (Ercolani, 1858) Hall, 1913

DH: MAN; domesticated cat and dog, and various species of wild canine and feline mammal

GD: The Americas (USA); Asia (Israel, Philippines); Oceania (Australia); helminth distributed in animal hosts worldwide

LM: Larval stage in skin; one case found by biopsy in skeletal muscle "... adult hookworm ... was recovered ... from the terminal colon ..."

ND: Cutaneous larva migrans due to *Ancylostoma caninum*. Ancylostomiasis due to *Ancylostoma caninum*

TM: Skin penetration by or ingestion of infective third-stage larva

Prociv, P. and Croese, J., 1990, Human eosinophilic enteritis caused by dog hookworm *Ancylostoma caninum*, **335**. *Lancet*, 1299-1302.

Ancylostoma ceylanicum (Looss, 1911) Leiper, 1915

DH: MAN; domesticated cat and dog and various species of wild feline mammal

GD: Asia (India, Japan, Malaysia, Taiwan). (Some localities doubtful due to problems of identification.)

LM: Adult in small intestine, larval stage migrates through tissues

ND: Ancylostomiasis due to *Ancylostoma ceylanicum*

TM: Ingestion of or skin penetration by infective third-stage larva

Carroll, S. M. and Grove, D. I., 1986, Experimental infections of humans with *Ancylostoma ceylanicum*: clinical, parasitological, haematological and immunological findings. *Tropical and Geographical Medicine*, **38**, 38-45.

Ancylostoma ceylanicum (Looss, 1911) Leiper, 1915

DH: MAN; occasionally in species of non-human primate, experimentally in domesticated cat and dog

GD: Worldwide (subtropical and warm temperate climate)

LM: Adult in small intestine, larval stage migrates through tissues

ND: Ancylostomiasis due to *Ancylostoma duodenale*.
Cutaneous larva migrans due to *Ancylostoma duodenale*

TM: Skin penetration by or ingestion of infective third-stage larva: transplacental and transmammary transmission possible

Hoagland, K. E. and Schad, G. A., 1978, *Necator americanus* and *Ancylostoma duodenale*: life history parameters and epidemiological implications of two sympatric hookworms of humans. *Experimental Parasitology*, **44**, 36-49.

Ancylostoma japonica Fukuda and Katsurada, 1925

DH: Man

GD: Asia (Japan)

LM: "... was reported once in man from Japan ... considered a species of doubtful validity"

TM: Presumably skin penetration by or ingestion of infective third-stage larva

Barriga, O. O., 1982, Ancylostomiasis. In *CRC Handbook Series in Zoonoses, Edited by J. H. Steele. Section C: Parasitic Zoonoses*, Volume II, edited by M. G. Schultz, (Boca Raton, Florida: CRC Press, Inc.), pp. 3-24.

Ancylostoma malayanum (Alessandrini, 1905)

DH: Man; usually found in bears

GD: Asia (Malaysia)

TM: Presumably skin penetration by or ingestion of third-stage larva

Yorke, W. and Maplestone, R. A., 1926, *The Nematode Parasites of Vertebrates.* (London: J. and A. Churchill). (See p. 93).

Ancylostoma tubaeforme Zeder, 1800

DH: Man; domesticated cat and other species of feline mammal

GD: Helminth widely distributed in feline hosts in temperate climates

LM: "Cutaneous larva migrans ... *Ancylostoma tubaeforme* ... may also be responsible"

TM: Presumably skin penetration by or ingestion of infective third-stage larva

Muller, R., 1975, *Worms and Disease* (London: William Heinemann Medical Books Ltd.). (See p. 87).

Bunostomum phlebotomum (Railliet, 1900)

DH: Man: domesticated cattle

GD: Helminth distributed in cattle worldwide

LM: Larval stage in skin

TM: Presumably skin penetration by infective third-stage larva

Beaver, P. C., Jung, R. C. and Cupp, E. W., 1984, *Clinical Parasitology*, 9th edition. (Philadelphia: Lea & Febiger), pp. 281-282.

Cyclodontostomum purvisi Adams, 1933

DH: Man; various species of rat

GD: Asia (Thailand)

LM: Presumably alimentary tract; "... the faecal specimen of a 47-year-old male patient ... was examined ... a pair of small unusual nematodes was recovered"

TM: Presumably accidental ingestion of infective third-stage larva on contaminated vegetables

Bhaibulaya, M. and Indrangarm, S., 1975, Man, an accidental host of *Cyclodontostomum purvisi* (Adams, 1933) and the occurrence in rats in Thailand. *Southeast Asian Journal of Tropical Medicine and Public Health*, **6**, 391-394.

Necator americanus (Stiles, 1902) Stiles 1903

DH: MAN; occasionally found in other species of mammal; experimentally in hamsters

GD: Worldwide (tropical and subtropical climates)

LM: Adult in small intestine, larval stage migrates through tissues

ND: Necatoriasis due to *Necator americanus*

TM: Skin penetration by infective third-stage larva

Migasena, S. and Gilles, H. M. 1987, Hookworm infection. *Bailliere's Clinical Tropical Medicine and Communicable Diseases*, 2, edited by Z. S. Pawlowski, (London and Philadelphia: Bailliere Tindall), pp. 617-627.

Necator argentinus Parodi, 1920

DH: Man

LM: "... has been reported once in man ...". (Possibly a synonym of *N. americanus*.)

TM: Presumably skin penetration by infective third-stage larva

Yoshida, Y., 1973, Species of hookworms infecting man: patterns of development. In *9th International Congress of Tropical Medicine and Malaria*. Abstract no. 255, Athens 174.

Necator suillus Ackert and Payne, 1922

DH: Man; domesticated pig

LM: "... human infection by the adult parasite has been attained at least once."

TM: Presumably skin penetration or ingestion of infective third-stage larva

Barriga, O. O., 1982, Ancylostomiasis. In *CRC Handbook Series in Zoonoses. Section C: Parasitic Zoonoses Volume II*, edited by M. G. Schultz, (Boca Raton, Florida: CRC Press, Inc.), pp. 3-24.

Uncinaria stenocephala (Railliet, 1884)

DH: Man; domesticated dog and species of small carnivorous mammal

GD: Helminth widely distributed in dogs in temperate climates

LM: Larval stage in skin

ND: Cutaneous larva migrans due to *Uncinaria stenocephala*

TM: Skin penetration by infective third-stage larva (usually ingestion of larva in dogs)

Bisseru, B., 1975, Cutaneous larva migrans, other Strongyloidea and Trichostrongyloidea. In *Diseases Transmitted from Animals to Man*, edited by W. T. Hubbert, W. F. McCulloch and P. R. Schnurrenberger (Springfield, Illinois: C. C. Thomas), pp. 611–619.

ANGIOSTRONGYLIDAE

Parastrongylus cantonensis (Chen, 1935)

S: *Angiostrongylus cantonensis*

DH: Man; rat and other species of rodent

IH: Species of snail and slug including *Achatina fulica* (terrestrial snail), *Pila scutata* (aquatic snail) and *Veronicella leydigi* (slug)

PH: *Birgus latra* (crab), *Hyla aurea* (frog) and *Macrobrachium lar* (shrimp)

GD: Africa (Ivory Coast); Asia (China, Indonesia, Japan, Malaysia, Taiwan, Thailand, Vietnam); The Americas (USA, Hawaii); Oceania (American Samoa, Vanuatu)

LM: Larval stage in brain, meninges and spinal cord

ND: Angiostrongyliasis due to *Parastrongylus cantonensis* or meningoencephalitis due to *Parastrongylus cantonensis*

TM: Ingestion of infective third-stage larva as a contaminant of vegetables or in undercooked intermediate and paratenic hosts

Cross, J. H., 1987, Public health importance of *Angiostrongylus cantonensis* and its relatives. *Parasitology Today*, **3**, 367–369.

Parastrongylus costaricensis Morera and Cespedes, 1971

S: *Angiostrongylus costaricensis*

DH: Man; *Sigmodon hispidus* (cotton rat) and other species of rodent

IH: *Vaginulus plebeius* (slug)

GD: The Americas (Costa Rica, Nicaragua, Panama, Peru)

LM: Adult in ileo-caeco-colic branches of the anterior mesenteric artery; occasionally liver and testicle.

ND: Angiostrongyliasis due to *Parastrongylus costaricensis*

TM: Ingestion of infective third-stage larva on vegetables contaminated by intermediate host

Morera, P., 1985, Abdominal angiostrongyliasis: a problem of public health. *Parasitology Today*, **1**, 173–175.

Parastrongylus mackerrasae Bhaibulaya, 1968

S: *Angiostrongylus mackerrasae*

DH: Man; species of rat

IH: Species of snail

GD: Helminth distributed in rodent hosts in Asia (Southeast Asia) and Oceania (Australia)

LM: "not parasitologically confirmed ... may be responsible for eosinophilic meningitis"

TM: Unresolved

Cross, J. H., 1987, Public health importance of *Angiostrongylus cantonensis* and its relatives. *Parasitology Today*, **3**, 367–369.

Parastrongylus malaysiensis Bhaibulaya and Cross, 1971

DH: Man

IH: Species of snail

GD: Asia (Southeast Asia); Oceania (Australia)

LM: "not parasitologically confirmed ... may be responsible for eosinophilic meningitis."

TM: Unresolved

Cross, J. H., 1987, Public health importance of *Angiostrongylus cantonensis* and its relatives. *Parasitology Today*, **3**, 367–369.

METASTRONGYLIDAE

Metastrongylus elongatus (Dujardin, 1844) Railliet and Henry, 1911

DH: MAN; domesticated and wild pig, various species of ruminant mammal

IH: *Lumbricus terrestris* and other species of earthworm

GD: Helminth distributed in domesticated pig and ruminants worldwide

LM: Respiratory tract

ND: Metastrongyliasis due to *Metastrongylus elongatus*

TM: Accidental ingestion of infective third-stage larva

Beaver, P. C., Jung, R. C. and Cupp, E. W., 1984, *Clinical Parasitology*, 9th edition. (Philadelphia: Lea & Febiger), pp. 291–292.

CHABERTIIDAE

Oesophagostomum aculeatum (Linstow, 1879)

DH: Man; species of non–human primate including *Macacus mulatta* (rhesus monkey), and species of ruminant

GD: Asia (Brunei, Indonesia)

LM: '... examination revealed a cutaneous lump ... was found to contain ... a worm.'

TM: Possibly skin penetration by infective larva

Ross, R. A., Gibson, D. I. and Harris, E. A., 1989, Cutaneous oesophagostomiasis in man. *Transactions of the Royal Society of Tropical Medicine and Hygiene*, **83**, 394–395.

Oesophagostomum apiostomum (Willach, 1891) Railliet and Henry, 1905

S: *Oesophagostomum brumpti*

DH: MAN; various species of non-human primate

GD: Africa (Togo)

LM: Adult worm attached to mucosa of large intestine, larval stage in tissue nodule associated with intestinal or abdominal wall

ND: Oesophagostomiasis due to *Oesophagostomum apiostomum*

TM: Accidental ingestion of infective third-stage larva

Dooley, J. R. and Neafie, R. C., 1976, Oesophagostomiasis. In *Pathology of Tropical and Extraordinary Diseases*, vol. 2, edited by C. H. Binford and D. H. Connor, (Washington D. C.: Armed Forces Institute of Pathology), pp. 440–445.

Oesophagostomum bifurcum (Creplin, 1849)

S: *Oesophagostomum apiostomum; O. brumpti*

DH: MAN; various species of non-human primate

GD: Africa (Ghana, Togo)

LM: Adult worm attached to mucosa of large intestine, larval stage in tissue nodule associated with intestinal or abdominal wall

ND: Oesophagostomiasis due to *Oesophagostomum bifurcum*

TM: Accidental ingestion of infective third-stage larva

Gigase, P., Baeta, S., Kumar, V. and Brandt, J., 1987, Frequency of symptomatic human oesophagostomiasis (Helminthoma) in Northern Togo. In *Helminth Zoonoses*, edited by V. Geerts, J. Kumart and J. Brandt, (Dordrecht, Boston and Lancaster: Martinus Nijhoff Publishers), pp. 228–236.

Oesophagostomum stephanostomum Railliet and Henry, 1909

DH: MAN; various species of non-human primate

GD: Africa (Ivory Coast); The Americas (Brazil)

LM: Adult worm attached to mucosa of large intestine, larval stage in tissue nodule associated with intestinal or abdominal wall

ND: Oesophagostomiasis due to *Oesophagostomum stephanostomum*

TM: Accidental ingestion of infective third-stage larva

Chabaud, A. G. and Lariviere, M., 1958, Sur les oesphagostomes parasites de l'homme. *Bulletin de la Societe de Pathologie Exotique*, **51**, 384–393.

Ternidens deminutus (Railliet and Henry, 1905) Railliet and Henry, 1909

DH: MAN; various species of non-human primate

IH: Unresolved

GD: Africa (Comoros, Malawi, Mauritius, Mozambique, South Africa, Tanzania, Uganda, Zaire, Zambia, Zimbabwe); helminth in non-human species of primate in Asia

LM: Adult worms in association with mucosa of large intestine, larval stages in tissue nodules in the large intestine

ND: Ternidensiasis

TM: Unresolved, may involve arthropod intermediate host

Goldsmid, J. M., 1982, *Ternidens* infection. In *CRC Handbook Series in Zoonoses. Section C. Parasitic Zoonoses*, II, edited by M. G. Schultz, (Boca Raton, Florida: CRC Press, Inc.), pp. 269–288.

SYNGAMIDAE

Mammomonogamus laryngeus (Railliet, 1899) Ryzhikov, 1948

S: *Syngamus laryngeus*

DH: MAN; various species of ruminant and feline mammal

GD: Africa (Cameroon, Central African Republic, Uganda); The Americas
(Argentina, Brazil, Colombia, Ecuador, Mexico, USA, Venezuela); Asia
(India, Malaysia, Philippines, Vietnam); The Caribbean (Saint Lucia,
Trinidad)

LM: Adult worm in air passage of upper respiratory tract

ND: Syngamiasis due to *Mammomonogamus laryngeus*

TM: Probably through ingestion of infective larva; an intermediate host may
be involved

Severo, L. C., Conci, L. M. A., Camargo, J. J. P., Andre-Alves, M. R. and Palombini, B. C.,
1988, Syngamosis: two new Brazilian cases and evidence of a possible pulmonary cycle.
Transactions of the Royal Society of Tropical Medicine and Hygiene, **82**, 467–468.

Mammomonogamus nasicola Buckley, 1934

S: *Syngamus nasicola*

DH: Man; species of herbivorous mammal including sheep, cattle, goat and
deer

GD: Caribbean (West Indies)

LM: "... 1913 pair of worms coughed up by woman in West Indies. (Identified by Leiper)"

TM: Presumably through ingestion of infective third-stage larva

Buckley, J. J. C., 1933, Some observations on two West Indian parasites of man.
Proceedings of the Royal Society of Medicine, **27**, 134–135.

TRICHOSTRONGYLIDAE

Haemonchus contortus (Rudolphi, 1803) Cobb, 1898

DH: MAN; domesticated ruminants and species of herbivorous mammal

GD: The Americas (Brazil); Asia (Iran); Oceania (Australia); helminth occurs frequently in domesticated ruminants worldwide

LM: Associated with the gastrointestinal mucosa

ND: Haemonchiasis

TM: Presumably through accidental ingestion of infective third-stage larva

Ghadirian, E. and Arfaa, F., 1973, First report of human infection with *Haemonchus contortus, Ostertagia ostertagi*, and *Marshallagia marshalli*, (family Trichostrongylidae) in Iran. *Journal of Parasitology*, **59**, 1144–1145.

Marshallagia marshalli (Ransom, 1907) Orlov, 1933

DH: MAN; domesticated ruminants and species of herbivorous mammal

GD: Asia (Iran); helminth widely distributed in animal hosts

LM: Associated with the gastrointestinal mucosa

TM: Presumably through accidental ingestion of infective larva

Ghadirian, E. and Arfaa, F., 1973, First report of human infection with *Haemonchus contortus, Ostertagia ostertagi*, and *Marshallagia marshalli*, (family Trichostrongylidae) in Iran. *Journal of Parasitology*, **59**, 1144–1145.

Mecistocirrus digitatus (von Linstow, 1906)

DH: MAN; various species of domesticated and wild ruminant and pig

GD: Helminth widely distributed in tropical countries

LM: Associated with the gastrointestinal mucosa

TM: Presumably through accidental ingestion of infective third-stage larva

Soulsby, E. J. L., 1982, *Helminths, Arthropods and Protozoa of Domesticated Animals*, 7th edition (London and Philadelphia: Bailliere Tindall). (See p. 238).

Nematodirus abnormalis May, 1920

DH: MAN; domesticated sheep and other species of herbivorous mammal

GD: Asia (Iran); helminth distributed in animal hosts in Asia, the Americas and Europe

LM: Alimentary tract; "After treatment with mebendazole one ... expelled two adult worms ... the other ... three adult worms ..."

TM: Presumably accidental ingestion of infective stage with contaminated herbage

Fallah, M., Taherkhani, H., Valadan, M. and Fashandaki, F., 1990, First report of human infection with *Nematodirus* sp. in Iran. *Bulletin de la Societe Francaise de Parasitologie*, **8**, Supplement 2, p. 892.

Ostertagia circumcincta (Stadlemann, 1894) Ransom, 1907

DH: MAN; domesticated goat and sheep and other species of ruminant

GD: Europe (USSR, Azerbaidjan); helminth widely distributed in animal hosts

LM: Associated with the gastrointestinal tract

TM: Presumably accidental, due to ingestion of nodular stage in under-cooked abomasum

Kasimov, B., 1943, First case of *Ostertagia ostertagi* in man in Azerbaidjan. *Medical Parasitology and Parasitic Diseases (Moscow)*, 12, 81. (This paper also describes a case of human infection with *O. circumcincta*.)

Ostertagia ostertagi (Stiles, 1892) Ransom, 1907

DH: MAN; domesticated cattle and other species of ruminant

GD: Asia (Iran); Europe (USSR, Azerbaidjan); helminth distributed in cattle worldwide

LM: Associated with the gastrointestinal tract

TM: Presumably accidental, due to ingestion of nodular stage in under-cooked abomasum

Kasimov, B., 1943, First case of *Ostertagia ostertagi* in man in Azerbaidjan. *Medical Parasitology and Parasitic Diseases (Moscow)*, 12, 81.

Trichostrongylus affinis Graybill, 1924

DH: MAN; rabbit and other species of herbivorous mammal

GD: Presumably related to that of rabbits

LM: Associated with the gastrointestinal tract

ND: Trichostrongyliasis due to *Trichostrongylus affinis*

TM: Presumably accidental ingestion of infective third-stage larva from contaminated herbage

Tongson, M. S. and Eduardo, S. L., 1982, Trichostrongylidosis. In *CRC Handbook Series in Zoonoses. Section C. Parasitic Zoonoses* Volume II, edited by M. G. Schultz, (Boca Raton, Florida: CRC Press, Inc.), pp. 331-337.

Trichostrongylus axei (Cobbold, 1879) Mennig, 1934

DH: MAN; domesticated and wild species of ruminant and herbivorous mammal, rabbits (experimental)

GD: Africa (Mauritius): Asia (Indonesia, Java; Japan); The Caribbean; Europe (USSR, Armenia, Siberia); Oceania (Australia)

LM: Associated with the gastrointestinal tract

ND: Trichostrongyliasis due to *Trichostrongylus axei*

TM: Presumably accidental ingestion of infective third-stage larva from contaminated herbage

Bundy, D. A. P., Terry, S. I., Murphy, C. P. and Harris, E. A., 1985, First record of *Trichostrongylus axei* infection of man in the Caribbean region. *Transactions of the Royal Society of Tropical Medicine and Hygiene*, **79**, 562–563.

Trichostrongylus brevis Otsuru, 1962

DH: MAN

GD: Asia (Japan)

LM: Alimentary tract; "... intestinal discharges ... following anthelmintic treatment ... worm was eliminated," (one male worm from each of three subjects)

ND: Trichostrongyliasis due to *Trichostrongylus brevis*

TM: Presumably by ingestion of infective third-stage larva from the contaminated environment

Otsuru, M., 1962, *Trichostrongylus brevis* sp. nov. from man (Nematoda: Trichostrongylidae). *Acta Medica et Biologica*, **9**, 273–278.

Trichostrongylus calcaratus Ransom, 1911

DH: MAN; rabbit, sheep and species of herbivorous mammal

GD: Asia (Iran)

LM: Associated with the gastrointestinal tract

ND: Trichostrongyliasis due to *Trichostrongylus calcaratus*

TM: Presumably accidental ingestion of infective third-stage larva from contaminated herbage

Biocca, E. and Paggi, L., 1959, Infestazione sperimentale di *Ovis aries* con larve di trichostrongili umani provenienti Dall'Iran. *Parassitologia*, **1**, 68–75.

Trichostrongylus capricola Ransom, 1907

DH: MAN; domesticated goat and sheep and other species of ruminant

GD: Asia (Iran); Europe (Italy)

LM: Associated with the gastrointestinal mucosa

ND: Trichostrongyliasis due to *Trichostrongylus capricola*

TM: Presumably accidental ingestion of infective third-stage larva from contaminated herbage

Ghadirian, E. and Arfaa, F., 1975, Present status of trichostrongyliasis in Iran. *American Journal of Tropical Medicine and Hygiene*, **24**, 935–941.

Trichostrongylus colubriformis (Giles, 1892) Ransom, 1911

DH: MAN; domesticated and wild species of ruminant and herbivorous mammal, guinea-pig (experimental)

GD: Africa (Egypt); The Americas (USA, Louisiana); Asia (India, Indonesia, Iran, Iraq, Japan); Europe (Italy; USSR, Armenia); Oceania (Australia); helminth widely distributed in species of domesticated ruminant

LM: Associated with the gastrointestinal tract

ND: Trichostrongyliasis due to *Trichostrongylus colubriformis*

TM: Presumably accidental ingestion of infective third-stage larva from contaminated herbage

Iori, A. and Cancrini, G., 1983, Indagini morfologiche comparative tra esemplari di *Trichostrongylus colubriformis* isolati da infestazioni umane e *T. colubriformis* da infestazioni sperimentali di *Ovis aries* con larve di provienza umana. *Parassitologia*, **25**, 17–20.

Trichostrongylus lerouxi Biocca, Chabaud and Ghadirian, 1974

DH: MAN; presumably species of domesticated ruminant

GD: Asia (Iran)

LM: Alimentary tract; "After anthelmintic treatment, stool specimens ... persons were harbouring *T. lerouxi*, ... "

ND: Trichostrongyliasis due to *Trichostrongylus lerouxi*

TM: Presumably accidental ingestion of infective third-stage larva from contaminated herbage

Ghadirian, F., 1977, Human infection with *Trichostrongylus lerouxi* (Biocca, Chabaud and Ghadirian, 1974) in Iran. *American Journal of Tropical Medicine and Hygiene*, **26**, 1212–1213.

Trichostrongylus orientalis Jimbo, 1914

DH: MAN; occasionally in species of domesticated ruminant

GD: Asia (China, Iran, Japan, Taiwan)

LM: Associated with the gastrointestinal tract

ND: Trichostrongyliasis due to *Trichostrongylus orientalis*

TM: Presumably accidental ingestion of infective third-stage larva from contaminated herbage

Biocca, E., Paggi, L. and Orecchia, P., 1960, Further studies on trichostrongyliasis in Jewish communities in Iran. *Parassitologia*, **1**, 345–352.

Trichostrongylus probolurus (Railliet, 1896) Looss, 1905

DH: MAN; domesticated and wild species of ruminant and herbivorous mammal

GD: Africa (Egypt); Asia (Iran); Europe (USSR, Armenia, Siberia)

LM: Associated with the gastrointestinal tract

ND: Trichostrongyliasis due to *Trichostrongylus probolurus*

TM: Presumably accidental ingestion of infective third-stage larva from contaminated herbage

Ghadirian, E. and Arfaa, F., 1975, Present status of trichostrongyliasis in Iran. *American Journal of Tropical Medicine and Hygiene*, **24**, 935–941.

Trichostrongylus skrjabini Kalantarian, 1930

DH: MAN; domesticated sheep and deer

GD: Asia (Iran); Europe (USSR, Armenia)

LM: Associated with the gastrointestinal tract

ND: Trichostrongyliasis due to *Trichostrongylus skrjabini*

TM: Presumably accidental ingestion of infective third-stage larva from contaminated herbage

Ghadirian, E. and Arfaa, F., 1975, Present status of trichostrongyliasis in Iran. *American Journal of Tropical Medicine and Hygiene*, **24**, 935–941.

Trichostrongylus vitrinus Looss, 1905

DH: MAN; domesticated and wild species of ruminant and herbivorous mammal

GD: Africa (Egypt, Morocco); The Americas (Chile); Asia (Iran); Europe (USSR, Armenia); helminth widely distributed in species of domesticated ruminant

LM: Associated with the gastrointestinal tract

ND: Trichostrongyliasis due to *Trichostrongylus vitrinus*

TM: Presumably accidental ingestion of infective third-stage larva from contaminated herbage

Poirriez, J., Dei-Cas, E., Guevart, E., Abdellatifi, M., Giard, P. and Vernes, A., 1984, Human infection with *Trichostrongylus vitrinus* in Morocco. *Annales Parasitologie Humaine et Comparee*, **59**, 636–639.

OXYURIDAE

Enterobius gregorii Hugot, 1983

DH: MAN

GD: Europe (France, U.K.)

LM: Caecum, appendix and colon

TM: Ingestion of egg containing infective larva

Chittenden, A. M. and Ashford, R. W., 1987, *Enterobius gregorii* Hugot, 1983; first report in the U.K. *Annals of Tropical Medicine and Parasitology*, **81**, 195–198.

Enterobius vermicularis (Linnaeus, 1758) Leach, 1853

S: *Oxyuris vermicularis*

DH: MAN; occasionally found in species of non-human primate

GD: Worldwide

LM: Associated with the mucosa and lumen of the caecum, appendix and colon

ND: Enterobiasis

TM: Ingestion (or inhalation) of egg containing infective larva

Marcus, L. C., 1982, Pinworm infections. In *CRC Handbook Series in Zoonoses, Section C. Parasitic Zoonoses* Volume II, edited by M. G. Schultz, (Boca Raton, Florida: CRC Press Inc.), pp. 251–253.

Syphacia obvelata (Rudolphi, 1802) Seurat, 1916

DH: MAN; mouse, other species of rodent and species of non–human primate

GD: Asia (Philippines); distributed worldwide in species of rodent

LM: Alimentary tract; " ... faecal sample ... from child ... eggs ... and two mature male ... worms."

TM: Presumably accidental ingestion of egg containing infective larva

Riley, W. A., 1920, A mouse oxyurid, *Syphacia obvelata*, as a parasite of man. *Journal of Parasitology*, **6**, 89–92.

ANISAKIDAE

Anisakis simplex (Rudolphi, 1809)

S: *Anisakis marina*

DH: Man; various species of piscivorous marine mammal

IH: *Thysanoessa longicaudata* and other species of euphausiid crustacean

PH: Species of marine fish and squid

GD: Asia (Japan); The Americas (USA); Europe (Baltic countries, Nether-lands, U.K.); helminth widely distributed in species of piscivorous marine mammal

LM: Associated with the wall of the stomach and small intestine

ND: Anisakiasis due to *Anisakis simplex*

TM: Ingestion of infective larva in raw or undercooked marine fish and squid

Oshima, T. and Klicks, M., 1986, Effects of marine mammal parasites on human health. In *Parasitology-Quo Vadit?* edited by M. J. Howell. Proceedings of the Sixth Internation-al Congress of Parasitology (Canberra: Australian Academy of Science), pp. 415–421.

Contracaecum osculatum Rudolphi (1802)

DH: Man; various species of piscivorous marine mammal and bird

IH: Species of euphausiid crustacean

PH: Species of marine fish

GD: Europe (Germany); helminth assumed to be widely distributed in species of piscivorous marine mammal

LM: Associated with the wall of the stomach and small intestine

ND: Anisakiasis due to *Contracaecum osculatum*

TM: Ingestion of infective larva in raw or undercooked marine fish

Williams, H. H. and Jones, A., 1976, Marine helminths and human health. *Commonwealth Institute of Helminthology, Miscellaneous Publication No.* 3, pp. 1–47.

Pseudoterranova decipiens (Krabbe, 1878)

DH: Man; various species of piscivorous marine mammal

IH: Species of marine crustacean

PH: Species of marine fish (and cephalopod)

GD: The Americas (Canada, USA); Asia (Japan)

LM: Associated with the wall of the stomach

ND: Anisakiasis due to *Pseudoterranova decipiens*

TM: Ingestion of infective larva in raw or undercooked marine fish (or cephalopod)

Oshima, T. and Klicks, M., 1986, Effects of marine mammal parasites on human health. In *Parasitology–Quo Vadit*? edited by M. J. Howell. Proceedings of the Sixth International Congress of Parasitology (Canberra: Australia Academy of Science), pp. 415–421.

ASCARIDIDAE

Ascaris lumbricoides Linnaeus, 1758

DH: MAN; occasionally in species of non-human primate and in dog, experimentally in pig; without complete development, in mouse, rabbit and species of laboratory mammal

GD: Worldwide

LM: Late larval and adult stage in lumen of the small intestine especially jejunum, early larval stage undertakes tissue migration through liver and lung

ND: Ascariasis due to *Ascaris lumbricoides*

TM: Ingestion of egg containing infective larva from food, water or contaminated environment generally

Crompton, D. W. T., 1989, Biology of *Ascaris lumbricoides*. In *Ascariasis and its Prevention and Control*, edited by D. W. T. Crompton, M. C. Nesheim and Z. S. Pawlowski, (London and Philadelphia: Taylor & Francis Ltd.), pp. 9–44.

Ascaris suum Goeze, 1782

DH: MAN; usually domesticated pig, experimentally in mouse, rabbit and laboratory animals, but with incomplete development

GD: Helminth distributed worldwide in countries where pigs are reared

LM: Late larval and adult stage in lumen of the small intestine, early larval stage undertakes tissue migration through liver and lung

ND: Ascariasis due to *Ascaris suum*

TM: Ingestion of egg containing infective larva from contaminated environment

Davies, N. J. and Goldsmid, J. M., 1978, Intestinal obstruction due to *Ascaris suum* infection. *Transactions of the Royal Society of Tropical Medicine and Hygiene*, **72**, 107.

Baylisascaris procyonis (Stefanski and Zarnowski, 1951)

DH: Man; *Procyon lotor* (raccoon)

GD: The Americas (USA); helminth widely distributed in raccoons

LM: Migrating larval stage reaches brain, lung, heart, intestinal tissue, lymph node

ND: Visceral larva migrans due to *Baylisascaris procyonis*

TM: Presumably accidental ingestion of egg containing infective larva from environment contaminated with raccoon faeces

Huff, D. S., Neafie, R. C., Binder, M. J., Guillermo, A., Brown, L. W. and Kazacos, K. R., 1984, Case 4. The first fatal *Baylisascaris* infection in humans: an infant with eosinophilic meningoencephalitis. *Pediatric Pathology*, **2**, 345–352.

Lagochilascaris minor Leiper, 1909

DH: MAN: usual hosts unresolved, presumably found in species of wild mammal

GD: The Americas (Brazil, Colombia, Costa Rica, Mexico, Surinam, Venezuela); The Caribbean (Trinidad and Tobago)

LM: Migrating larval stage found in subcutaneous abscess (neck, ear, mastoid process, orbit, paranasal sinus, retropharingeal tissue); egg-producing adult found in subcutaneous abscess and in lung in one case.

TM: Presumably accidental ingestion of egg containing infective larva from contaminated environment

Moraes, M. A. P., Arnaud, M. V. C., de Macedo, R. C. and Anglada, A. E., 1985, Infeccao pulmonar fatal por *Lagochilascaris* sp., provavelemente *Lagochilascaris minor*, Leiper, 1909. *Revista do Instituto de Medicina Tropical de Sao Paulo*, **27**, 46–52.

Parascaris equorum (Goeze, 1782) Yorke and Maplestone, 1926

DH: Man; domesticated horse and other species of equine mammal

GD: Helminth distributed worldwide in species of equine mammal

LM: Visceral larval migrans and pneumonitis

TM: Ingestion of egg containing infective larva from contaminated environment

Bisseru, B., 1975, *Ascaris* and visceral larval migrans. In *Diseases Transmitted from Animals to Man*, 6th edition, edited by W. T. Hubbert, W. F. McCulloch and P. R. Schnurrenberger, (Illinois: Charles C. Thomas), pp. 584–600.

Toxascaris leonina (von Linstow, 1902) Leiper, 1907

DH: Man; domesticated cat and dog, species of wild felidae and canidae

GD: Helminth widely distributed in species of cat and dog

LM: Adult stage found in small intestine; migrating larval stage assumed to occur in deeper parts of the body

ND: Visceral larva migrans due to *Toxascaris leonina*

TM: Presumably accidental ingestion of egg containing infective larva from contaminated environment

Leiper, R. T., 1907, Two new genera of nematodes occasionally parasitic in man. *British Medical Journal*, **1**, 1296–1298.

Toxocara canis (Werner, 1782) Johnston, 1916

DH: Man, may occasionally attain sexual maturity; usually found in domesticated dog and related species of mammal

GD: Worldwide in countries where dogs are reared

LM: Migrating larval stage occurs in deeper parts of the body, invasion of the eye may occur; "... to produce an adult specimen of *T. canis* in a child aged 16 months ... " (Galliard, 1974, In *Parasitic Zoonoses* ed. E. J. L. Soulsby, [New York: Academic Press], pp. 295–304.)

ND: Visceral larval migrans due to *Toxocara canis*; endophthalmitis due to *Toxocara canis* (if ocular involvement diagnosed)

Glickman, L. and Schantz, P. M., 1981, Epidemiology and pathogenesis of zoonotic toxocariasis. *Epidemiological Review*, **3**, 230–250.

Toxocara cati (Schrank, 1788) Brumpt, 1927

DH: Man, may attain sexual maturity; usually found in domesticated cat and related species of mammal

GD: Worldwide in countries where cats are reared

LM: Migrating larval stage occurs in deeper parts of the body; adult in alimentary tract, worms have been passed in stool and vomites and one female with eggs has been recovered from a child's anus.

ND: Visceral larva migrans due to *Toxocara cati*

TM: Ingestion of egg containing infective larva from contaminated environment

Beaver, P. C., Jung, R. C. and Cupp, E. W., 1984, *Clinical Parasitology*, 9th edition. (Philadelphia: Lea & Febiger), (See pp. 325–328).

Toxocara pteropodis Baylis, 1936

DH: Man; helminth usually found in *Pteropus geddier* and *P. poliocephalus* (fruit bats)

GD: Oceania (Vanuatu)

LM: Larval stage assumed to be involved with the liver*

TM: Presumably accidental ingestion of egg containing infective larva from contaminated environment

Moorhouse, D. E., 1982, Toxocariasis: a possible cause of Palm Island Mystery Disease. *Medical Journal of Australia*, **1**, 172–173.

*Palm Island Mystery Disease was described by Byth (1980: *Medical Journal of Australia*, **2**, 40–42) following an outbreak of a disease with hepatitis-like symptoms in 1979 in a community from Palm Island, Vanuatu. Prociv (1989: *Parasitology Today*, **5**, 106–109) suggests poisoning with copper sulphate was the cause of Palm Island Mystery Disease.

Toxocara vitulorum (Goeze, 1782) Travassos, 1927

DH: Man; domesticated bovines and other species of ruminant mammal

GD: Helminth distributed worldwide in countries where cattle are reared

LM: Possible cause of visceral larva migrans

TM: Presumably accidental ingestion of egg containing infective larva; transmammary route involved in animal hosts

Van Gorp, K., Mangelschots, M. and Brandt, J., 1987, *Toxocara vitulorum*: a possible agent of larva migrans in humans? In *Helminth Zoonoses*, edited by S. Geerts, V. Kumar and J. Brandt, (Dordrecht, Boston, Lancaster: Martinus Nijhoff Publishers), pp. 159–166.

DRACUNCULIDAE

Dracunculus medinensis (Linnaeus, 1758) Gallandant, 1773

DH: MAN; domesticated dog and other species of carnivorous and herbivorous mammal including species of non-human primate

IH: Species of freshwater copepod (Crustacea) including *Cyclops leuckarti* and other species of *Cyclops*, *Eucyclops* and *Macrocyclops*

GD: Predominantly in the Northern Hemisphere in arid and semiarid countries of Africa and Asia.

LM: Larval stage migrates through the body, adult worm found in subcutaneous tissue

ND: Dracunculiasis

TM: Ingestion of freshwater contaminated with copepod containing infective third-stage larva

Muller, R., 1971, *Dracunculus* and dracunculiasis. *Advances in Parasitology*, **9**, 73–151.

PHILOMETRIDAE

Philometra sp. Costa, 1845

DH: Man; usually found in species of marine fish including *Caranx melampygus* (jackfish)

IH: Species of marine copepod (Crustacea)

GD: The Americas (USA, Hawaii)

LM: "A female (adult) dracunculoid, *Philometra* sp., invaded a puncture wound in a fisherman's hand while he was filleting an infected carangid fish."

TM: Accidental transfer from fish host

Deardorff, T. L., Overstreet, R. M., Okihiro M. and Tam, R., 1986, Piscine adult nematode invading an open lesion in a human hand. *American Journal of Tropical Medicine and Hygiene*, **35**, 827–830.

GNATHOSTOMATIDAE

Gnathostoma doloresi Tubangui, 1925

DH: Man; domesticated and wild pig

IH1:   Species of freshwater copepod including *Cyclops vicinus, Eucyclops serrulatus* and *Mesocyclops leuckarti*

IH2/PH: *Oncorhynchus masou* (brook trout); various species of amphibian and reptile known to harbour infective third-stage larva

GD: Asia (Japan); helminth distributed in pigs in India, Malaysia and the Philippines

LM: Larval stage in skin; " ... were able to detect parasites in the biopsied skin samples of 3 out of 7 cases."

ND: Gnathostomiasis due to *Gnathostoma doloresi*

TM: Presumably ingestion of infective larva from either first or second intermediate or paratenic host

Ogata, K., Imai, J. I. and Nawa, Y., 1988, Three confirmed and five suspected human cases of *Gnathostoma doloresi* infection found in Miyazaki Prefecture, Kyushu. *Japanese Journal of Parasitology*, **37**, 358–364.

Gnathostoma hispidum Fedtschenko, 1872

DH: Man; domesticated and wild pig

IH1: Species of *Cyclops* (copepod)

IH2: Various species of freshwater fish including *Misgurnus anguillicaudatus* (loach) and species of amphibian and mammal

GD: Asia (China, India); helminth widely distributed in countries where pigs are reared.

LM: Helminth found in the eye in one case in China

ND: Gnathostomiasis due to *Gnathostoma hispidum*

TM: Presumably ingestion of infective larva from either first or second intermediate host

Chen, H. T., 1949, A human ocular infection by *Gnathostoma* in China. *Journal of Parasitology*, **35**, 431–433.

Gnathostoma spinigerum Owen, 1836

DH: Man, may attain sexual maturity; domesticated cat and dog, various species of wild carnivorous mammal

IH1: Species of freshwater copepod including *Cyclops leuckarti* and *Eucyclops serrulatus*

IH2: Species of freshwater crayfish and fish, species of amphibian, reptile, mammal and domesticated fowl

GD: The Americas (Mexico; USA, California); Asia (Bangladesh, Cambodia, India, Indonesia, Japan, Laos, Malaysia, Myanmar, Philippines, Thailand, Vietnam)

LM: " ... the infection is characterized by migratory swellings, subcutaneous larva migrans or abscesses which are usually peripheral but occasionally involve the eyes, lungs, abdomen or brain."

ND: Gnathostomiasis due to *Gnathostoma spinigerum*

TM: Ingestion of infective larva in one of the many species of second intermediate host that form items of human diets; evidence of prenatal transmission in one case.

Radomyos, P. and Daengsvang, S., 1987, A brief report on *Gnathostoma spinigerum* specimens from human cases. *Southeast Asian Journal of Tropical Medicine and Hygiene*, **18**, 215–217.

PHYSALOPTERIDAE

Physaloptera caucasica von Linstow, 1902

DH: MAN; species of non-human primate

IH: Unresolved, presumably species of beetle and/or cockroach (second intermediate host and/or paratenic host may be involved)

GD: Africa (Zaire, Zambia, Zimbabwe); The Americas (Brazil, Colombia, Panama); Asia (India, Israel)

LM: Alimentary tract

ND: Physalopteriasis

TM: Presumably accidental ingestion of infective larva

Hira, P. R., 1976, Observations on helminth zoonoses in Zambia. *East African Medical Journal*, **53**, 278–286.

Physsaloptera transfuga Marits and Grinberg, 1970

DH: Man; domesticated cat and dog, species of amphibian and reptile

IH: Probably species of beetle

GD: Europe (USSR)

LM: ". .. specimens of *Physaloptera transfuga* n.sp. recovered from the lower lip of a woman in Moldavia, U.S.S.R.".

TM: Presumably accidental contact with infective larva

Marits, N. M. and Grinberg, A. Z., 1970, *Physaloptera transfuga* n.sp. (Nematoda, Physalopteridae). In [*Parasites of Animals and Plants*] Kishinev: RIO Akad. Nauk. Moldavskoi SSR **5**, 67–72. *Helminthological Abstracts*, **40**, 4675.

RICTULARIIDAE

Rictularia sp. Froelich, 1802

DH: MAN; species of rodent and bat

IH: Presumably species of arthropod

GD: The Americas (USA, New York)

LM: "A gravid female nematode was found in histopathologic sections of an appendix in a *post mortem* examination."

TM: Presumably accidental ingestion of intermediate host containing infective larva

Kenny, M., Eveland, L. K., Vermakov, V. and Kassouny, D. Y., 1975, A case of *Rictularia* infection of man in New York. *American Journal of Tropical Medicine and Hygiene*, **24**, 596–598.

THELAZIIDAE

Thelazia californiensis Price, 1930

DH: Man; domesticated cat and dog, various species of wild mammal

IH: Species of dipteran flies including *Fannia benjamini* (canyon fly) and *Musca autumnalis* (face fly)

GD: The Americas (USA, California)

LM: ". .. resident . .. had a slightly red eye . .. showed marked follicular hypertrophy of the ... conjunctiva. On everting the upper lid a round-worm was found in the upper culdesac."

ND: Thelaziasis due to *Thelazia californiensis*

TM: Introduction of infective larva into the orbit as dipteran intermediate host feeds on eye secretions

Lee, R. D. and Parmelee, W. E., 1958, Thelaziasis in man. *American Journal of Tropical Medicine and Hygiene*, **7**, 427–428.

Thelazia callipaeda Railliet and Henry, 1910

DH: MAN; domesticated dog, various species of mammal

IH: Species of dipteran flies including *Phortina variegata*

GD: Asia (China, India, Japan, Korea, Myanmar); Europe (USSR)

LM: "Eight adult worms ... removed from the conjunctival sac of a ... woman ..."

ND: Thelaziasis due to *Thelazia callipaeda*

TM: Introduction of infective larva into orbit as dipteran intermediate host feeds on eye secretions

Adachi, K. and Sato, H., 1988, A case of *Thelazia callipaeda* infection in human conjunctival sac in Tottori Prefecture, Japan. *Ganka Rinsyouihou*, **82**, 228–231.

GONGYLONEMATIDAE

Gongylonema pulchrum Molin, 1857

DH: MAN; species of domesticated ruminant, pig, horse and camel

IH: Species of coprophagous beetle; experimentally in *Blatella germanica* (cockroach)

GD: Africa (Morocco); The Americas (USA); Asia (China, Sri Lanka); Europe (Spain); Oceania (Australia, New Zealand)

LM: Larval and adult stages in mucosa and submucosa of the buccal cavity

ND: Gongylonemiasis due to *Gongylonema pulchrum*

TM: Accidental ingestion of intermediate host containing infective larva

Illescas-Gomez, M. P., Osario, M. R., Garcia, V. G. and Morales, M. A. G., 1988, Human *Gongylonema* infection in Spain. *American Journal of Tropical Medicine and Hygiene*, **38**, 363–365.

SPIROCERCIDAE

Spirocerca lupi (Rudolphi, 1809)

DH: MAN; domesticated dog, various species of wild canine and feline mammal

IH: Species of coprophagous beetle including *Scarabeus sacer*

GD: Europe (Italy); helminth widely distributed in dogs

LM: "Adults ... embedded in pockets of the terminal ileum."

TM: Assumed transplacental migration from mother to foetus in this specific case, the mother having ingested the infective third-stage larva in the intermediate host

Biocca, E., 1959, Infestazione umana prenatale da *Spirocerca lupi* (Rud., 1809). *Parassitologia*, **1**, 137–142.

ACUARIIDAE

Cheilospirura sp. Diesing, 1861

ND: Conjunctivitis due to *Cheilospirura* sp.

TM: Accidental ingestion of intermediate host containing infective larva

GD: Asia (Philippines); *Cheilospirura hamulosa* is widely distributed in species of domesticated poultry

LM: Eye

ND: Conjunctivitis due to *Cheilospirura* sp.

TM: Accidental ingestion of intermediate host containing infective larva

Africa, C. M. and Garcia, E. Y., 1936, A new nematode parasite (*Cheilospirura* sp.) of the eye of man in the Philippines. *Journal of the Philippine Islands Medical Association,* **16,** 603–607.

FILARIOIDEA

ONCHOCERCIDAE

Wuchereria bancrofti (Cobbold, 1877) Seurat, 1921

DH: MAN; *Presbytis cristatus* (leaf monkey, experimental)

IH: Many species of mosquito including *Aedes poicilius, Anopheles barbirostris* and *Culex quinquefasciatus*

GD: Many tropical and subtropical countries

LM: Sheathed microfilariae found in blood (usually nocturnal), adults in lymphatics

ND: Filariasis due to *Wuchereria bancrofti*

TM: Introduction of infective third-stage larva when female mosquito takes a blood meal

Ciba Foundation Symposium 127, 1987, *Filariasis*. (Chichester, New York, Toronto, Singapore: John Wiley and Sons), 305 pp.

Wuchereria lewisi Schacher, 1969

DH: MAN*

IH: Mosquito

GD: The Americas (Brazil)

LM: Sheathed microfilariae found in blood

TM: Introduction of infective larva when female mosquito takes a blood meal

Schacher, J. F., 1969, Intraspecific variation in microfilariae with description of *Wuchereria lewisi* sp. nov. (Nematoda, Filaroidea) from man in Brazil. *Annals of Tropical Medicine and Parasitology*, **63**, 341–351.

Brugia beaveri Ash and Little, 1964

DH: MAN; *Lynx rufus* (bobcat), *Mustela vison* (mink) and *Procyon lotor* (raccoon)

IH: *Aedes aegypti* (mosquito, experimental)

GD: The Americas (USA, Louisiana)

LM: "A mature male worm ... found in ... an enlarged, painful retroauricular lymph node ..."

TM: Presumably, introduction of infective larva when intermediate host takes a blood meal

Schlesinger, J. J., Dubois, J. G. and Beaver, P. C., 1977, *Brugia*-like filarial infection acquired in the United States. *American Journal of Tropical Medicine and Hygiene*, **26**, 204–207.

*Adult worm assumed to be present because microfilariae were observed.

Brugia guyanensis Orihel, 1964

DH: MAN; *Nasua nasua* (coatamundi)

IH: Unresolved

GD: The Americas (Peru)

LM: "... adult male worm and gravid female worm ... in a lymphatic vessel of a right cervical lymph node."

TM: Presumably introduction of infective larva when intermediate host takes a blood meal

Baird, J. K. and Neafie, R. C., 1988, South American brugian filariasis: Report of a human infection acquired in Peru. *American Journal of Tropical Medicine and Hygiene*, **39**, 185–188.

Brugia malayi (Brug, 1927) Buckley, 1958

DH: MAN; species of non-human primate including *Macaca irus* (crab-eating macaque), species of cat and *Manis javanica* (pangolin)

IH: Species of *Aedes*, *Anopheles* and *Mansonia* (mosquitoes)

GD: Asia (Indonesia, Malaysia, Philippines, Thailand, Vietnam)

LM: Sheathed microfilariae found in blood, adults in lymphatics

ND: Filariasis due to *Brugia malayi*

TM: Introduction of infective third-stage larva when female mosquito takes a blood meal

Dissanaike, A. S., 1986, A review of *Brugia* sp. with special reference to *Brugia malayi* and to zoonotic infections. *Tropical Biomedicine*, **3**, 67–72.

Brugia pahangi (Buckley and Edeson, 1956)

DH: MAN (experimental); domesticated cat and dog, various species of mammal

IH: Species of mosquito including *Anopheles barbirostris* and *Mansonia* spp (natural) and species of *Aedes, Anopheles, Armigeres, Culex* and *Psorophora* (experimental)

GD: Asia (Western Malaysia)

LM: Presumably sheathed microfilariae found in blood, adults in lymphatics

TM: Experimentally, infective larva inoculated subcutaneously.

Edeson, J. F. B., Wilson, T., Wharton, R. H. and Laing, A. B. G., 1960, Experimental transmission of *Brugia malayi* and *B. pahangi* to man. *Transactions of the Royal Society of Tropical Medicine and Hygiene*, **54**, 229–234.

Brugia timori Partono, Purnomo, Dennis, Atmosoedjono, Oemijati and Cross, 1977

DH: MAN; *Meriones unguiculatus* (Mongolian jird, experimental)

IH: Species of mosquito including *Anopheles barbirostris* (natural) and *Aedes togoi* (experimental)

GD: Asia (Indonesia, Lesser Sunda Islands)

LM: Sheathed microfilariae found in blood (nocturnal), adults in lymphatics

ND: Filariasis due to *Brugia timori*

TM: Introduction of infective third-stage larva when female mosquito takes a blood meal

Partono, F., Purnomo, A., Dennis, D. T., Atmosoedjono, S., Oemijati, S. and Cross, J. H., 1977, *Brugia timori* sp.n. (Nematoda: Filarioidea) from Flores Island, Indonesia. *Journal of Parasitology*, **63**, 540–546.

Onchocerca volvulus (Leuckart, 1893) Railliet and Henry, 1910

DH: MAN; non-human species of primate including *Ateles geoffroy* (spider monkey), *Gorilla gorilla* (gorilla), *Pan satyrus* (chimpanzee, experimental)

IH: Species of blackfly (Diptera) including *Simulium damnosum* complex, *S. neavei* (Africa and Asia); *S. callidum, S. exiguum, S. metallicum, S. ochraceum* (The Americas)

GD: Africa (27 countries in tropical region); The Americas (Brazil, Colombia, Ecuador, Guatemala, Mexico, Venezuela); Asia (Yemen);

LM: Unsheathed microfilariae found in skin and eye, adults in palpable nodules

ND: Onchocerciasis

TM: Introduction of infective third-stage larva when blackfly takes a blood meal

W.H.O., 1987, *Onchocerciasis.* Report of a W.H.O. Expert Committee. *Technical Report Series* No. 752 (Geneva: World Health Organization).

Mansonella (M) *ozzardi* (Manson, 1897) Faust, 1929

DH: MAN

IH: Species of Diptera including *Culicoides furens* and *Simulium amazonicum*

GD: The Americas (Argentina, Bolivia, Brazil, Colombia, French Guyana, Mexico, Panama, Peru, Venezuela); The Caribbean (Anguilla, Antigua, Dominica, Dominican Republic, Guadeloupe, Haiti, Martinique, St Lucia, St Vincent)

LM: Unsheathed microfilariae found in blood, adults in body cavities frequently embedded in the mesenteries

ND: Mansonelliasis due to *Mansonella ozzardi*

TM: Introduction of infective third-stage larva when insect takes a blood meal

Godoy, G. A., Volcan, G., Medrano, C., Teixeira, A. and Matheus, L., 1980, *Mansonella ozzardi* infections in Indians of the southwestern part of the state of Bolivar, Venezuela. *Americal Journal of Tropical Medicine and Hygiene*, **29**, 373–376.

Mansonella (Esslingeria) ***perstans*** (Manson, 1891) Orihel and Eberhard, 1982

S: *Dipetalonema perstans*

DH: MAN; species of non-human primate including *Pan satyrus* (chimpanzee)

IH: Species of *Culicoides* (midges)

GD: Africa (widespread); The Americas (East-coast countries of S. America); The Caribbean (Trinidad)

LM: Unsheathed microfilariae found in blood, adults in peritoneal cavity, kidney region and hepatic portal tissue

ND: Mansonelliasis due to *Mansonella perstans*

TM: Introduction of infective third-stage larva when insect takes a blood meal

Baird, J. K., Neafie, R. C., Lanoie, L. and Connor, D. H., 1987, Adult *Mansonella perstans* in the abdominal cavity of nine Africans. *American Journal of Tropical Medicine and Hygiene*, **37**, 578–584.

*Mansonella **semiclarum*** Fain, 1974

DH: MAN*

IH: Unresolved

GD: Africa (Zaire)

*Adult worm not yet described from human host, but assumed to be present because microfilariae were observed

LM: Unsheathed mircofilariae found in blood

TM: Presumably introduction of infective third-stage larva when intermediate host takes a blood meal

Dujardin, J. P., Fain, A. and Maertens, K., 1982, Survey on the human filariasis in the
region of Bwamanda in Northwest Zaire. *Annales de la Societe Belge de Medecine
Tropicale*, **62**, 315–342.

Mansonella (Esslingeria) streptocerca (Macfie and Corson, 1922) Orihel and
Eberhard, 1982

S: *Dipetalonema streptocerca*

DH: MAN; species of non-human primate including *Gorilla gorilla* (gorilla)
and *Pan troglodytes* (chimpanzee)

IH: Species of *Culicoides* (midges)

GD: Africa (Congo, Ghana, Zaire)

LM: Unsheathed microfilariae in skin, adults in subcutaneous tissue

ND: Mansonelliasis due to *Mansonella streptocerca*

TM: Introduction of infective third-stage larva when insect takes a blood
meal

Meyers, W. M., Neafie, R. C., Moris, R. and Bourland, J., 1977, Streptocerciasis:
observation of adult male *Dipetalonema streptocerca* in man. *American Journal of
Tropical Medicine and Hygiene*, **26**, 1153–1155.

Dipetalonema arbuta Highby, 1943

DH: Man; "... identified as possibly *D. arbuta* from *Erethizon dorsatum*
(porcupine) or *D. sprenti* from *Castor canadensis* (beaver)"

IH: Species of *Aedes* (mosquitoes)

GD: The Americas (USA, Oregon)

LM: "... a parasite was removed from the eye ..."

TM: Presumably introduction of infective third-stage larva when insect takes a blood meal

Orihel, T. C., 1985, Filariae. In *Animal Agents and Vectors of Human Disease*, 5th edn., edited by P. C. Beaver and R. C. Jung, (Philadelphia; New York and London), p. 190.

Dipetalonema sprenti Anderson, 1953

DH: Man; "... identified as possibly *D. arbuta* from *Erethizon dorsatum* (porcupine) or *D. sprenti* from *Castor canadensis* (beaver)"

IH: Species of *Aedes* (mosquitoes)

GD: The Americas (USA, Oregon)

LM: "... a parasite was removed from the eye ..."

TM: Presumably introduction of infective third-stage larva when insect takes a blood meal

Beaver, P. C., Meyer, E. A., Jarroll, E. L. and Rosenquist, R. C., 1980, *Dipetalonema* from the eye of a man in Oregon, U.S.A. A case report. *American Journal of Tropical Medicine and Hygiene*, **29**, 369–372.

Microfilaria bolivarensis Godoy, Orihel and Volcan, 1980

DH: MAN*

IH: Unresolved

GD: The Americas (Bolivia, Venezuela)

*Adult worm not yet described from human host, but assumed to be present because mircofilariae were observed

LM: Unsheathed microfilariae found in blood

TM: Presumably introduction of infective third-stage larva when intermediate host takes a blood meal

Godoy, G. A., Orihel, T. C. and Volcan, G. S., 1980, *Microfilaria bolivarensis:* a new species of filaria from man in Venezuela. *American Journal of Tropical Medicine and Hygiene*, **29**, 545-547.

Microfilaria (Mansonella) rodhaini Peel and Chardome, 1974

DH: MAN*; *Pan paniscus* and *P. satyrus* (chimpanzees)

IH: Possibly species of *Culicoides* (midges)

GD: Africa (Gabon)

LM: Unsheathed microfilariae found in skin

TM: Presumably introduction of infective third-stage larva when intermediate host takes a blood meal

Richard-Lenoble, D., Kombila, M., Bain, O., Chandenier, J. and Mariotte, O., 1988, Filariasis in Gabon: human infections with *Microfilaria rodhaini*. *American Journal of Tropical Medicine and Hygiene*, **39**, 91–92.

Meningonema peruzzii Orihel and Esslinger, 1973

DH: MAN*; species of monkey including *Cercopithecus talapoin* (talapoin monkey)

IH: Unresolved

GD: Africa (Equatorial Guinea, Uganda, Zimbabwe)

LM: Sheathed microfilariae found in cerebrospinal fluid

---

*Adult worm not yet described from human host, but assumed to be present because microfilariae were observed.

ND: Meningonemiasis

TM: Presumably introduction of infective third-stage larva when intermediate host takes a blood meal

Orihel, T. C., 1973, Cerebral filariasis in Rhodesia – a zoonotic infection? *American Journal of Tropical Medicine and Hygiene*, **22**, 596–599.

Setaria equina (Abildgaard, 1789)

DH: Man; domesticated camel, cattle and horse

IH: Species of culicidae (midges)

GD: Asia (India); worldwide in species of domesticated equine mammal

LM: Unresolved

TM: Presumably introduction of infective larva when insect takes a blood meal

Gupta, N. K. and Kalia, D. C., 1978, On nematodes of some live-stock animals in India. *Revista Iberia Parasitologia*, **38**, 35–61.

Dirofilaria (D) immitis (Leidy, 1856) Railliet and Henry, 1911

DH: Man; domesticated cat and dog, various species of wild carnivorous mammal

IH: Species of *Aedes*, *Anopheles* and *Culex* (mosquitoes)

GD: The Americas (USA, Brazil, Colombia); Asia (Japan); Oceania (Australia); helminth widely distributed in dogs in tropical, subtropical and warm temperate regions of the world.

LM: "… in man, however, the cycle is arrested and the sexually immature nematode is embolized to the lung."

ND: Dirofilariasis due to *Dirofilaria immitis*

TM: Introduction of infective third-stage larva when female mosquito takes a blood meal

Larrieu, A. J., Wiener, M. D., Gomez, L. G. and Williams, E. H., 1979, Human pulmonary dirofilariasis presenting as a solitary pulmonary nodule. *Chest*, **75**, 511–512.

Dirofilaria (Nochtiella) repens Railliet and Henry, 1911

DH: Man, may attain sexual maturity; domesticated cat and dog, various species of wild carnivorous mammal

IH: Species of *Aedes* and *Anopheles* (mosquitoes)

GD: Africa (Unresolved, probably Nigeria); Asia (Israel, Sri Lanka); Europe (France, Greece, Italy, USSR, Yugoslavia); helminth widely distributed in dogs

LM: "... individuals with 2 mobile subcutaneous nodules ..."

ND: Dirofilariasis due to *Dirofilaria repens*

TM: Introduction of infective third-stage larva when female mosquito takes a blood meal

Carneri, I. de, Sacchi, S. and Pazzaglia, A., 1973, Subcutaneous dirofilariasis in man – not so rare. *Transactions of the Royal Society for Tropical Medicine and Hygiene*, **67**, 887–888.

Dirofilaria spectans Freitas and Lent, 1949

DH: Man; *Pteronura brasiliensis* (Giant otter)

IH: Unresolved

GD: The Americas (Brazil)

LM: "Diagnosis of arterial obstruction was made by ... arteriography and surgical retreat of the parasite."

TM: Introduction of infective third-stage larva when intermediate host takes a blood meal

Teixeira de Freitas, J. F. and Mayall, R., 1953, Fenomeno de Raynaud na mao esquerda provocado por *Dirofilaria spectans*. *Revista Brasileira de Medicina*, **10**, 463–467.

Dirofilaria (Nochtiella) striata (Molin, 1858)

DH: Man; various species of wild cat

IH: *Anopheles quadrimaculatus* (mosquito, experimental)

GD: The Americas (USA, North Carolina)

LM: Presumably adults in subcutaneous tissue

ND: Dirofilariasis due to *Dirofilaria (Nochtiella) striata*

TM: Presumably introduction of infective third-stage larva when female mosquito takes a blood meal

Orihel, T. C. and Beaver, P. C., 1974, Zoonotic filariasis in the United States. *Proceedings of the 3rd International Congress of Parasitology* **B 13**(45), p. 651.

Dirofilaria (Nochtiella) tenuis Chandler, 1942

DH: MAN; *Procyon lotor* (raccoon)

IH: *Aedes taeniorhyncus, Anopheles quadrimaculatus* and *Psorophora confinis* (mosquitoes)

GD: The Americas (USA, Florida, Mississippi, N. Carolina)

LM: Adults and immature worms in subcutaneous tissue particularly in the orbital area. "The worm had ... reproductive duct containing spermatozoa."

ND: Dirofilariasis due to *Dirofilaria (Nochtiella) tenuis*

TM: Presumably introduction of infective third-stage larva when female mosquito takes a blood meal

Font, R. L., Neafie, R. C. and Perry, H. D., 1980, Subcutaneous dirofilariasis of the eyelid and ocular adnexa. Report of six cases. *Archives of Ophthalmology*, **98**, 1079–1082.

Dirofilaria (Nochtiella) ursi Yamaguti, 1941

DH: Man; various species of bear including *Ursus torquatus japonicus*

IH: Species of *Simulium* including *S. venustrum* (blackfly)

GD: The Americas (Canada, USA); helminth widely distributed in bears in Japan, Canada and northern USA

LM: "The worm, an infertile female ... was removed in a subcutaneous nodule ..."

ND: Dirofilariasis due to *Dirofilaria (Nochtiella) ursi*

TM: Presumably introduction of infective third-stage larva when blackfly takes a blood meal

Beaver, P. C. and Samuel, W. M., 1977, Dirofilariasis in man in Canada. *American Journal of Tropical Medicine and Hygiene*, **26**, 329-330.

Loa loa (Cobbold, 1864) Castellani and Chalmers, 1913

DH: MAN; species of non-human primate including *Cercopithecus nictitans* (putty-nose monkey) and *Mandrillus leucophaeus* (drill)

IH: Species of *Chrysops* including *C. dimidiata* and *C. silacea* (tabanid flies)

GD: Africa (from Senegal in the West to the Sudan in the East)

LM: Sheathed microfilariae found in blood (diurnal), adults in subcutaneous tissue (provoke Calabar swelling) and may pass under the conjunctiva found in the eye.

ND: Loiasis

TM: Introduction of infective third-stage larva when female tabanid takes a blood meal

Hawking, F., 1977, The distribution of human filariasis throughout the world. Part III. Africa. *Tropical Diseases Bulletin*, 74, 650-679.

NEMATOMORPHA

GORDIIDAE

Gordius aquaticus Linnaeus, 1758

H: Man; free-living adult worm in fresh water after development in the body cavity of insect

GD: The Americas (El Salvador); Europe (Germany, Italy, Romania, Switzerland, U.K., Yugoslavia); worm widely distributed

LM: Presumably alimentary tract; worms known to be vomited and passed per rectum

TM: Unresolved

Zschokke, F. von, 1912, *Gordius aquaticus* as a parasite of man. *Science* n.s. **35**, 636.

Gordius chilensis Blanchard, 1849

H: Man; free-living adult worm in fresh water after development in the body cavity of insect

GD: The Americas (Chile)

LM: Presumably alimentary tract

TM: Unresolved

Cappucci, D. T., 1976, The biology of *Gordius robustus* Leidy with a host list and summary of the public health importance of the Gordioidea. *PhD Thesis*, University of California, San Francisco. 77-7789. University Microfilm, Ann Arbor, Michigan 48106, U.S.A.

Gordius gesneri Heinze, 1937

H: Man; free-living adult worm in fresh water after development in the body cavity of insect

GD: Europe (Germany)

LM: Presumably alimentary tract; male specimen, vomited by a female patient

TM: Unresolved

Heinze, K., 1937, Die Saitenwurmer (Gordioidea) Deutschlands. Eine systematisch-faunistiche Studie uber Insektenparasiten aus der Gruppe der Nematomorpha. *Zeitschrift fur Parasitenkunde*, **9**, 263-344.

Gordius inesae Cavalieri, 1961

H: Man; free-living adult worm in fresh water after development in the body cavity of insect

GD: The Americas (Argentina)

LM: Presumably alimentary tract; male specimen recovered from the vomitus of a woman

TM: Unresolved

Cavalieri, F., 1961, Descripcion de una neuva especie de Gordiaces *Gordius inesae* n. sp. (Gordioidea, Gordiidae). *Neotropica*, **7**, 3-6.

Gordius ogatai

H: Man; free-living adult worm in fresh water after development in the body cavity of species of insect

GD: Asia (Japan)

LM: Presumably alimentary tract; "... worms were vomited ... were discharged per anus."

TM: Unresolved

Uchikawa, R., Akune, K., Tinoue, I., Kagei, N. and Sato, A., 1987, A human case of hair worm (*Gordius* sp.) infection in Kagoshima, Japan. *Japanese Journal of Parasitology*, **36**, 358-360.

Gordius perronciti Camerano, 1897

H: Man; free-living adult worm in fresh water after development in the body cavity of insect

GD: Europe (Germany)

LM: Presumably alimentary tract; worms known to be vomited

TM: Unresolved

Heinze, K., 1937, Die Saitenwurmer (Gordioidea) Deutschlands. Eine systematisch-faunistische studie uber Insektenparasiten aus der Gruppe der Nematomorpha. *Zeitschrift fur Parasitenkunde*, **9**, 263-344.

Gordius reddyi Singh and Rao, 1966

H: Man; free-living adult worm in fresh water after development in the body cavity of insect

GD: Asia (India)

LM: Four specimens described from a tumorous mass in the orbit of a patient in India.

TM: Unresolved

Singh, S. N. and Rao, V. G., 1966, On a case of human infection with a gordiid worm in the orbit. *Indian Journal of Helminthology*, **18**, (Senior Supplement), pp. 65-67.

Gordius robustus Leidy, 1851

H: Man; free-living adult worm in fresh water after development in the body cavity of insect

GD: The Americas (USA, Florida, Utah)

LM: Encapsulated in the lower eyelid and passed from the urethra

TM: Possibly from drinking water contaminated with infective larval stage

Sayad, W. Y., Johnson, V. M. and Faust, E. C., 1936, Human parasitization with *Gordius robustus*. *Journal of the American Medical Association*, **106**, 461-462.

Gordius setiger Schneider, 1866

H: Man; free-living adult worm in fresh water after development in the body cavity of insect

GD: Europe

TM: Unresolved

Faust, E. C., Russell, P. F. and Jung, R. C., 1970, Nematomorpha. In *Craig and Faust's Clinical Parasitology*, eighth edition. (Philadelphia: Lea & Febiger), pp. 405-406.

Gordius skorikowi Camerano, 1903

H: Man; free-living adult worm in fresh water after development in the body cavity of insect

GD: Asia (Sri Lanka)

LM: Presumably alimentary tract; male specimen from the vomitus of a 3-year-old boy

TM: Unresolved

Fernando, C. H. and Dissanaike, A. S., 1962, A hairworm (Gordiacea) "parasitic" in a child in Ceylon. *Ceylon Journal of Medical Science*, **11**, 47-49.

CHORDODIDAE

Chordodes capensis, Camerano 1895

H: Man; free-living adult worm in fresh water after development in the body cavity of insect

GD: Africa (Tanzania)

LM: "... female specimen ... passed (? per anum) ..."

TM: Unresolved

Baylis, H. A., 1927, Notes on two gordiids and a mermithid said to have been parasitic in man. *Transactions of the Royal Society of Tropical Medicine and Hygiene,* **21,** 303-306.

Neochordodes colombianus Faust and Botero, 1960

H: Man; free-living adult worm in fresh water after development in the body cavity of insect

GD: The Americas (Colombia)

LM: External meatus of the ear

TM: Unresolved

Faust, E. C. and Botera, R. D., 1960, Extraordinario hallazgo de una nueva especie de Neochordodes (Gordiacea) en Colombia. *Homenaje al Dr Eduardo Cabellero y Caballero, Mexico,* D.F. p. 523-527.

Parachordodes alpestris (Villot, 1884)

H: Man; free-living adult worm in fresh water after development in the body cavity of insect

GD: Europe (France)

LM: Presumably alimentary tract; female specimen vomited

TM: Unresolved

Gueguen, F., 1905, Sur un nouveau cas de parasitisme occasionnel dans le tube digestif de l'homme, d'un nematode du genre *Gordius* Dujardin. *Bulletin Scientifique Pharmacologie*, **12**, 257-266.

Parachordodes pustulosus Baird, 1853

H: Man; free-living adult worm in fresh water after development in the body cavity of insect

GD: Europe (Italy)

LM: Presumably alimentary tract; worm passed per anum

TM: Unresolved

Parona, C., 1901, Altra caso di pseudo-parassitismo di gordio nell'uomo (*Parachordodes pustulosus* Baird). *Clinica Medical Italiana*, **40**, 627-632.

Parachordodes raphaelis (Camerano, 1893)

H: Man; free-living adult worm in fresh water after development in the body cavity of insect

GD: Africa (South Africa)

LM: "... passed per urethrum."

TM: Unresolved

Yeh, Liang-Sheng and Jordan, P., 1957, A new gordiid worm parasitic in man. *Annals of Tropical Medicine and Parasitology*, **51**, 313-316.

Parachordodes tolosanus (Dujardin, 1842)

H: Man; free-living adult worm in fresh water after development in the body cavity of insect

GD: Europe (France)

LM: Presumably alimentary tract; worms known to be vomited and passed per anum

TM: Unresolved

Degland, C. D., 1821, Observation sur un ver filiforme rendu par le vomissement. *Memoires de la Societe d' emulation de Cambrai*, **6**, 204-211.

Parachordodes violaceus (Baird, 1853)

H: Man; free-living adult worm in fresh water after development in the body cavity of insect

GD: Europe (France)

LM: Presumably alimentary tract; worm known to be vomited

TM: Unresolved

Topsent, E., 1900, Sur un cas de pseudoparasitisme chez l'homme du *Gordius violaceus* Baird. *Bulletin de la Societe des Sciences Naturelles de L'Ouest de La France*, **9**, 86-91.

Parachordodes wolterstorffii (Camerano, 1888)

H: Man; free-living adult worm in fresh water after development in the body cavity of insect

GD: Europe (U.K.)

LM: "... specimen passed per vaginum ..."

TM: Unresolved, but possibly from use of water, contaminated with larval stage, as a vaginal douche

Baylis, H. A., 1944, Notes on the distribution of hairworms (Nematomorpha: Gordiidae) in the British Isles. *Proceedings of the Zoological Society of London Series B*, **113** (1943), 193-197.

Paragordius areolatus von Linstow, 1906

H: Man; free-living adult worm in fresh water after development in the body cavity of insect

GD: Africa (Ghana)

LM: "Two adult female Gordiids ... passed by a girl"

TM: Unresolved

Baylis, H. A., 1927, Notes on two gordiids and a mermithid said to have been parasitic in man. *Transactions of the Royal Society of Tropical Medicine and Hygiene*, **21**, 203-206.

Paragordius cinctus von Linstow, 1906

H: Man; free-living adult worm in fresh water after development in the body cavity of species of insect

GD: Africa (South Africa , Transvaal)

LM: Presumably alimentary tract

TM: Unresolved

Linstow, von, 1906, Gordiiden und Mermithiden des Koniglechen. Zoologischen Museums in Berlin. *Mitteilungen aus dem Zoologischen Museum in Berlin*, **3**, 241-248.

Paragordius esavianus Carvalho, 1942

H: Man; free-living adult worm in fresh water after development in the body cavity of insect

GD: The Americas (Brazil)

LM: "... was expelled by girl through urethra ..."

TM: Unresolved

Carvalho, J. C. M., 1942, Studies on some Gordiacea of North and South America. *Journal of Parasitology*, **28**, 213-222.

Paragordius tricuspidatus (Dufour, 1828)

H: Man; free-living adult worm in fresh water after development in the body cavity of insect

GD: Europe (France)

LM: Vomited from throat of 15-year-old French boy

TM: Unresolved

Blanchard, R., 1897, Pseudo-parasitisme d'un *Gordius* chez l'homme. *Bulletin de L'Academie Nationale de Medecine (Paris)*, **37**, 614-618.

Paragordius varius (Leidy, 1851)

H: Man; free-living adult worm in fresh water after development in the body cavity of insect

GD: The Americas (Canada)

LM: "... passing per anum ... 'large quantities' of *Paragordius varius* (Leidy) on two occasions 1 week apart." Also per urethra.

TM: Unresolved, but "The worm was probably ingested by drinking unfiltered well water"

Ali-Khan, F. E. A. and Ali-Khan, Z., 1977, *Paragordius varius* (Leidy) (Nematomorpha) infection in man: a case report from Quebec (Canada). *Journal of Parasitology*, **63**, 174-175.

Pseudogordius tanganyikae Yeh and Jordan, 1957

H: Man; free-living adult worm in fresh water after development in the body cavity of insect

GD: Africa (Tanzania)

LM: Adult female worm " ... was passed, it is believed per urethrum ... although possibly passed per rectum."

TM: Unresolved

Yeh, L. S. and Jordan, P., 1957, A new gordiid worm parasitic in man. *Annals of Tropical Medicine and Parasitology*, **51**, 313-316.

ACANTHOCEPHALA

ARCHIACANTHOCEPHALA

MONILIFORMIDAE

Moniliformis moniliformis (Bremser, 1811) Travassos, 1915

DH: MAN; species of rodent especially *Rattus norvegicus* and *R. rattus*

IH: Species of insect including *Periplaneta americana* (cockroach) and *Geotrupes impressus* (beetle)

PH: *Bufo marinus* (toad), *Ctenosaura* sp. (lizard)

GD: Occasional infections of humans are known from a number of countries worldwide

LM: Small intestine

ND: Acanthocephaliasis due to *Moniliformis moniliformis*

TM: Ingestion of insect intermediate host containing cystacanth

Al-Rawas, Y. A., Mirza, Y. M. and Shafiq, M. A., 1977, First finding of *Moniliformis moniliformis* (Bremser, 1811) Travassos, 1915 (Acanthocephala: Oligocanthorhynchidae) in Iraq from a human child. *Journal of Parasitology*, **63**, 396-397.

OLIGACANTHORHYNCHIDAE

Macracanthorhyncus hirudinaceus (Pallas, 1781) Travassos, 1917

DH: MAN; domesticated and wild pig

IH: Species of insect including *Cotinus nitida*, *Dorysthenes paradoxus* and *Popillia japonica* (beetles) and *Periplaneta americana* (cockroach)

GD: Africa (Madagascar); Asia (China); Europe (USSR); sporadic reports of the helminth from humans in other locations

LM: Small intestine

ND: Acanthocephaliasis due to *Macracanthorhynchus hirudinaceus*

TM: Ingestion of intermediate host containing cystacanth

Zhong, H-L., Feng, L-B., Wang, C-X., Kang, B., Wang, Z-Z., Zhou, G-H., Zhao, Y. and Zhang, Y-Z., 1983, Human infection with *Macracanthorhynchus hirudinaceus* causing serious complications in China. *Chinese Medical Journal*, **96**, 661-668.

Macracanthorhynchus ingens (von Linstow, 1879) Meyer, 1932

DH: MAN; *Procyon lotor* (raccoon), *Mephitis mesomelas* (skunk) and other species of carnivorous mammal

IH: Terrestrial arthropods, *Parcoblatta pensylvanica* (woodroach) and *Narceus americanus* (millipede)

PH: Various species of frog and snake

GD: The Americas (USA, Texas); helminth distributed widely in *Procyon lotor* (raccoon)

LM: Small intestine

ND: Acanthocephaliasis due to *Macracanthorhyncus ingens*

TM: Presumably accidental ingestion of intermediate host containing cystacanth or paratenic host containing juvenile

Dingley, D. and Beaver, P. C., 1985, *Macracanthorhynchus ingens* from a child in Texas. *American Journal of Tropical Medicine and Hygiene*, **34**, 918-920.

PALAEACANTHOCEPHALA

ECHINORHYNCHIDAE

Acanthocephalus rauschi (Schmidt, 1969) Golvan, 1969

DH: Man; possibly species of marine fish

IH: Probably species of marine Crustacea

PH: Unresolved

GD: The Americas (USA, Alaska)

LM: Peritoneum

ND: Acanthocephaliasis due to *Acanthocephalus rauschi*

TM: Presumably by ingestion of cystacanth in intermediate host or possibly juvenile encysted in paratenic host (undercooked fish)

Golvan, Y. J., 1969, Systematique des acanthocephales (Acanthocephala, Rudolphi, 1801). Premiere partie L'ordre des Echinorhynchoidea (Cobbold 1876), Golvan et Houin 1963. *Memoires du Museum National d'Histoire Naturelle*, **47**, 1-373.

Pseudoacanthocephalus bufonis (Shipley, 1903) Petrotshenko, 1958

DH: Man; *Bufo melanostictus* and other species of toad

IH: Unresolved presumably species of arthropod

PH: Unresolved

GD: Asia (Indonesia, Java); helminth widely distributed in species of Amphibia in Asia

LM: Small intestine

ND: Acanthocephaliasis due to *Pseudoacanthocephalus bufonis*

TM: Presumably ingestion of intermediate host containing cystacanth or paratenic host containing juvenile

Lie-Kian Joe and Tan Kok Siang, 1959, Human intestinal helminths obtained from autopsies in Djakarta, Indonesia. *American Journal of Tropical Medicine and Hygiene*, **8**, 518-523.

POLYMORPHIDAE

***Bolbosoma* sp. Porta, 1908**

DH: Man; helminths of this genus infect species of Cetacea

IH: Probably species of marine Crustacea

PH: Probably species of marine fish

GD: Asia (Japan)

LM: " ... jejunum ... purulent material ... 2-cm-long worm ..."

ND: Acanthocephaliasis due to *Bolbosoma* sp.

TM: Possibly ingestion of juvenile in raw or undercooked fish

Tado, I., Otsuji, Y., Kamiya, H., Mimori, T., Sakaguchi, Y. and Makizumi, S., 1983, The first case of a human infected with an acanthocephalan parasite, *Bolbosoma* sp. *Journal of Parasitology*, **69**, 205-208.

***Corynosoma strumosum* (Rudolphi, 1802) Lühe, 1904**

DH: Man; species of seal

IH: Probably species of marine amphipod (Crustacea)

PH: Various species of brackish water and marine teleost fish

GD: The Americas (USA, Alaska)

LM: "It was found in a stool ... after treatment with atabrine."

ND: Acanthocephaliasis due to *Corynosoma strumosum*

TM: Presumably ingestion of juvenile in raw or undercooked fish

Schmidt, G. D., 1971, Acanthocephalan infections of man with two new records. *Journal of Parasitology*, **57**, 582-584.

SUMMARY TABLES

Distribution by major taxa of the numbers of species of
helminth recorded from human hosts

Helminth taxa		Number of species	
Platyhelminthes	Turbellaria	3	
	Digenea	113	173
	Eucestoda	57	
Nematoda		138	
Nematomorpha		24	
Acanthocephala		7	
		342	

Distribution by major taxa of the host status and helminth site of numbers of species of helminth recovered from human hosts

	Host status[a]				Helminth site[b]			
Helminth taxa[c]	Definitive	Intermediate	Paratenic	Undefined	Alimentary tract	Cavities, organs and tissues	Skin and tissues	Circulatory system
P. Turbellaria	–	–	–	3	2	1	–	–
P. Digenea	83	1	2	29	68	32	25	9
P. Eucestoda	38	14	–	6	44	15	–	–
NEMATODA	69	3	–	67	61	51	31	12
NEMATOMORPHA	–	–	–	24	16	7	–	–
ACANTHOCEPHALA	3	–	–	4	6	1	–	–
	193	18	2	133	197	107	56	21

[a] Host status (see pp. 20 and 21) is assigned on the basis of an assessment of published information from a variety of sources. In some cases, e.g. *Taenia solium* (p. 112), humans serve as both intermediate and definitive hosts.

[b] The sites in which helminths have been found or appear to live in human hosts. *Alimentary tract* (buccal cavity to anus) includes the biliary system and pancreatic duct. *Cavities, organs and tissues* includes the CNS, excretory, respiratory and reproductive systems, muscles, lymphatics and deep body tissues; helminths involved in visceral larva migrans are shown under this heading. *Skins and tissues* is shown for helminths that are involved in cutaneous larva migrans and skin penetration followed by tissue migration as well as for helminths that live in the skin. *Circulatory system* is restricted to the heart and blood vessels. Many species of helminth occupy more than one site in the human body during the host-parasite relationship; *Ascaris lumbricoides* (p. 153) undergoes an extensive tissue migration and an intestinal phase. In some cases, reliable information about a helminth's site is not readily available.

[c] P, Platyhelminthes

Index